Doctor, What's The Alternative?

Also by Dr Hilary Jones

BEFORE YOU CALL THE DOCTOR

YOUR CHILD'S HEALTH

I'M TOO BUSY TO BE STRESSED

Doctor, What's The Alternative?

Everything you need to know about complementary therapies – what's available and what *really* works

Dr Hilary Jones

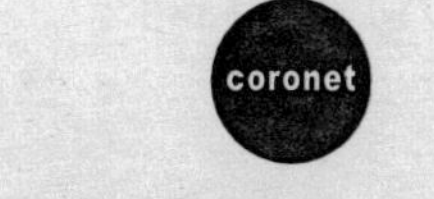

CORONET BOOKS
Hodder & Stoughton

First published in Great Britain in 1998 by Hodder & Stoughton
A division of Hodder Headline PLC

A Coronet paperback

10 9 8 7 6 5 4 3 2 1

A CIP catalogue record for this title is available from the British Library.

ISBN 0 340 72827 2

Printed and bound in Great Britain by
Mackays of Chatham plc, Chatham, Kent

Hodder and Stoughton
A Division of Hodder Headline PLC
338 Euston Road
London NW1 3BH

To my family
and to all patients everywhere
who remain uncertain
about their treatment

Contents

ACKNOWLEDGEMENTS

[illegible]

I should also like to acknowledge [illegible] from the progressive [illegible] Marylebone Health [illegible] in London and the Hall [illegible] for Complementary [illegible] not a stone's throw from [illegible] Regent's Park. I thank too [illegible] Yates and Patrice Clark for [illegible] help in researching the text.

Acknowledgements

I should first like to thank all those thousands of people I have seen over the years as patients whose experiences of complementary medicine and whose questions relating to the subject have stimulated, intrigued or stunned me.

I should also like to thank my tutors at the Royal Free Hospital Medical School who gave me an excellent grounding in orthodox and scientific medicine whilst still allowing me to retain an enquiring and open mind about less scientific but traditional 'alternative' therapies.

In particular I should like to thank Linda Tagg for teaching me the rudiments of acupuncture, Dr Keith Bush for encouraging me to incorporate osteopathy into my general practice, and the late Dr Charles Cohen for demonstrating to me for the first time the fascinating and therapeutically powerful technique of hypnosis. Through the integration of these complementary procedures into my allopathic medical repertoire, I have come to appreciate how much some of the 'alternative therapies' can offer.

I would also like to thank Rowena Webb, my editor, for demonstrating so clearly the need for such a book and for persuading me that I was the right person to write it. I thank Sarah, my wife, for patiently deciphering my doctor's handwriting and typing the manuscript, and Dr Brenda Davies for sharing with me her unique and charismatic ability to mix formal psychotherapy with spiritual healing and other holistic remedies to the everlasting benefit of her patients.

I should also like to acknowledge the help I received from the progressive and excellent Marylebone Health Centre in London and the Hale Clinic for Complementary Therapy not a stone's throw from it off Regent's Park. I thank too David Yates and Farine Clark for their help in researching the book.

Finally, a special word of thanks to all those therapists, teachers and experts in their various complementary fields who freely and willingly contributed so generously to Part Two of the book, and to all those patients who happily communicated their frank opinions on the complementary therapies they had experienced by doing likewise. They are:

D. Allum, Jafe Arif, Mary Bennett, Bonnie Blowers, Claudine Bowman, Sandy Brice, Gemma Bridges, Sue Cleasby, Dr Brenda Davies, Mark Devene, Mary Dollan, Colin Douglas, Enid A. Eden, Elizabeth Fraser, Edward Gartland, Lesley Goodman, J. Hallum, David Hankin, Nigel Alan Hartley, Judith Hayes, Matthew Hemmings, B. Hennessy, Mary Chase Hopkins, Adam J. Jackson, Vega John, Nic Kyriacou, Gordon K. Linscott, Beth MacEoin, Anne Miller, Dana Morgan, Margaret O'Malley, Barbara Nagle, Linda Powell, Gary Prosser, Andrea Richards, A. Robbins, Kim Sawyer, Jennifer Smith, Phillippa Stacy, Barbara Stanhope-Williamson, Maryon Stewart, Linda A. Tagg, Bren Taylor, Mary Timms, Garry Trainer, R. Newman Turner, Patsy Wendle, Mark White, David Whitton, Dr Peter J. Whorwell, Nicholas Woodhead, David Yates.

I'm very grateful to them all.

A N

Throughout thi
'complementary
terms 'orthodox
Some definitio
'complementary
of and a substitu
mentary medicin
therapy is somet
conjunction with
In reality, the
blurred. There ar
medical care. A w
mastectomy opera
combination radio
the same time tal
aromatherapist w
hospital bed, and s
yoga classes or tryi
medical care wher
therapies are blend
satisfactory integra
definitions of alter
no more than an ex
in everyday parla
medicine as one an
regarded throughou

Introduction

More and more patients are asking about alternatives to conventional medical treatments suggested to them by their doctors. This is only to be welcomed. It is also the over-riding reason for writing this book. As a National Health Service family doctor who has trained in a number of complementary therapies, and incorporated them into his daily working life, including nutritional therapy, osteopathy, acupuncture and hypnotherapy, I am acutely aware of how useful these and other practices can be. I realize, too, how rewarding they can prove for both therapist and patient alike. But I'm also aware of the massive confusion about alternative medicine that uncritical media coverage has often brought about. Outrageous claims are made for its apparent benefits, while at the same time well-proven, established, conventional medical practices are rubbished or dismissed.

Orthodox medicine is powerful. It can certainly save lives in critical situations, but in less acute circumstances it also has the ability to produce serious side effects, and it can create iatrogenic diseases, that is illnesses caused by doctors themselves (see page 41), and a complete disempowerment and passivity within patients. Alternative medicine, on the other hand, is gentler, and at the same time allows the patient much greater responsibility for his or her own health. It should never be considered for life-threatening situations such as meningitis, diabetes or appendicitis, but for the vast majority of ailments and symptoms experienced by people who wish to feel better, it offers a tremendous potential for physical, emotional and spiritual support. For the chronic diseases like rheumatoid arthritis and strokes, where traditional doctors all too often throw in the towel, alternative medicine is a crutch. For all those stress-related problems, such as migraine, palpitations and irritable bowel syndrome, it is a comfort. For those controversial disorders associated with our polluted modern environment, like ME (myalgic encephalomyelitis), attention deficit hyperactivity disorder, asthma and food intolerance, it is a tonic. For emotional and psychological difficulties, such as anxiety, depression and panic attacks, it is a godsend. For the large proportion of patients who see their doctor for non-specific or vague symptoms which do not fit into any neat or convenient category of recognized disease, it offers choice. To the thousands of people who, by dint of their lifestyles, have never realized their full potential for good health and fitness, it shows a new way forward. And finally, for all those who wish desperately to find some help with coming to terms with disability or even terminal illness whilst remaining in control of their own destiny, alternative medicine promises hope and preservation of the spirit.

Alternative medicine can therefore achieve many things. But there is also much it cannot achieve. It, too, has its limitations. Contrary to popular belief it is not always safe, natural, free of side effects and successful. Much of it is unregulated, its practitioners a law unto themselves and its benefits over-exaggerated and scientifically unproven. It also costs patients time and money. How can people make sense of it all? How do they decide which therapist they should take their symptoms to, and which of the various treatments would be appropriate for them? Never before has a full and proper answer to the question, 'Doctor, what's the alternative?' been so badly needed. This book, I hope, provides that answer.

PART ONE

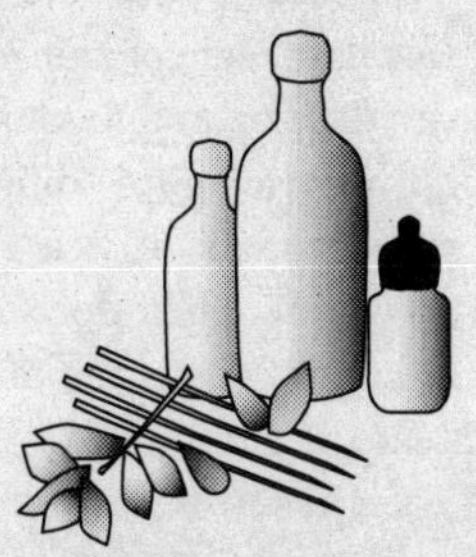

Complementary Versus Orthodox Medicine

Acknowledgements

I should first like to thank all those thousands of people I have seen over the years as patients whose experiences of complementary medicine and whose questions relating to the subject have stimulated, intrigued or stunned me.

I should also like to thank my tutors at the Royal Free Hospital Medical School who gave me an excellent grounding in orthodox and scientific medicine whilst still allowing me to retain an enquiring and open mind about less scientific but traditional 'alternative' therapies.

In particular I should like to thank Linda Tagg for teaching me the rudiments of acupuncture, Dr Keith Bush for encouraging me to incorporate osteopathy into my general practice, and the late Dr Charles Cohen for demonstrating to me for the first time the fascinating and therapeutically powerful technique of hypnosis. Through the integration of these complementary procedures into my allopathic medical repertoire, I have come to appreciate how much some of the 'alternative therapies' can offer.

I would also like to thank Rowena Webb, my editor, for demonstrating so clearly the need for such a book and for persuading me that I was the right person to write it. I thank Sarah, my wife, for patiently deciphering my doctor's handwriting and typing the manuscript, and Dr Brenda Davies for sharing with me her unique and charismatic ability to mix formal psychotherapy with spiritual healing and other holistic remedies to the everlasting benefit of her patients.

I should also like to acknowledge the help I received from the progressive and excellent Marylebone Health Centre in London and the Hale Clinic for Complementary Therapy not a stone's throw from it off Regent's Park. I thank too David Yates and Farine Clark for their help in researching the book.

Finally, a special word of thanks to all those therapists, teachers and experts in their various complementary fields who freely and willingly contributed so generously to Part Two of the book, and to all those patients who happily communicated their frank opinions on the complementary therapies they had experienced by doing likewise. They are:

D. Allum, Jafe Arif, Mary Bennett, Bonnie Blowers, Claudine Bowman, Sandy Brice, Gemma Bridges, Sue Cleasby, Dr Brenda Davies, Mark Devene, Mary Dollan, Colin Douglas, Enid A. Eden, Elizabeth Fraser, Edward Gartland, Lesley Goodman, J. Hallum, David Hankin, Nigel Alan Hartley, Judith Hayes, Matthew Hemmings, B. Hennessy, Mary Chase Hopkins, Adam J. Jackson, Vega John, Nic Kyriacou, Gordon K. Linscott, Beth MacEoin, Anne Miller, Dana Morgan, Margaret O'Malley, Barbara Nagle, Linda Powell, Gary Prosser, Andrea Richards, A. Robbins, Kim Sawyer, Jennifer Smith, Phillippa Stacy, Barbara Stanhope-Williamson, Maryon Stewart, Linda A. Tagg, Bren Taylor, Mary Timms, Garry Trainer, R. Newman Turner, Patsy Wendle, Mark White, David Whitton, Dr Peter J. Whorwell, Nicholas Woodhead, David Yates.

I'm very grateful to them all.

A Note About Terminology

Throughout this book, the terms 'alternative medicine' and 'complementary medicine' are used interchangeably, as are the terms 'orthodox medicine' and 'conventional medicine'.

Some definitions seek to distinguish between 'alternative' and 'complementary', suggest that alternative medicine is exclusive of and a substitute for conventional medicine, whereas complementary medicine, although still being a totally distinct form of therapy is something which can be used happily alongside, in conjunction with, and complementary to orthodox practice.

In reality, the boundaries of all these types of therapy are blurred. There are alternative treatments even within conventional medical care. A woman with cancer of the breast may decline a mastectomy operation in favour of the alternative approach of combination radiotherapy and hormone treatment. She might at the same time take advantage of a visit from a reflexologist or aromatherapist whilst she remains an in-patient in an NHS hospital bed, and she may also derive benefit from attending some yoga classes or trying some herbal preparations to complement her medical care when she gets home. For someone like her, all the therapies are blended together into an all-encompassing and highly satisfactory integrated model of health care. Precise and esoteric definitions of alternative and complementary medicine are really no more than an exercise in futile tautology. I believe most people in everyday parlance regard alternative and complementary medicine as one and the same thing, so this is how they have been regarded throughout this book.

Foreword by Uri Geller

At a time when alternative medicine is growing so fast in popularity and when the limitations of conventional medicine are being so widely publicized, it is essential that a reliable, well-researched and objective account of what alternative medicine can and cannot achieve is available.

So much hype surrounds the promise and attraction of alternative medicine but much of it is anecdotal or unscientific. Just because something is natural does not necessarily mean it is safe, and just because a therapy derives from some mystical ancient folklore does not necessarily mean we can abandon the orthodox trappings of modern clinical medicine. We would only do that at our peril.

But my own insight and experience into that which defies ordinary explanation – events which are by definition *extra-ordinary* – but which are nevertheless tangible, real and reproducible, direct me to embrace the magic and mysticism of alternative medical therapies. I myself have benefited from some of them in numerous ways.

Dr Hilary Jones' book is responsible, informative, realistic and utterly balanced. This is only what I would expect from someone I have come to know and work with, and who has earned such a well-recognized and established medical reputation. He also practises several kinds of complementary therapies himself, such as acupuncture, osteopathy and hypnosis. Anyone expressing an interest in exploring alternative solutions to their physical, psychological or emotional problems would do very well to read this book before they go any further.

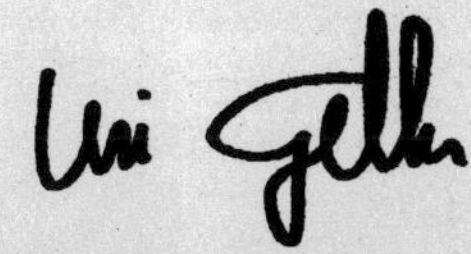

Introduction

More and more patients are asking about alternatives to conventional medical treatments suggested to them by their doctors. This is only to be welcomed. It is also the over-riding reason for writing this book. As a National Health Service family doctor who has trained in a number of complementary therapies, and incorporated them into his daily working life, including nutritional therapy, osteopathy, acupuncture and hypnotherapy, I am acutely aware of how useful these and other practices can be. I realize, too, how rewarding they can prove for both therapist and patient alike. But I'm also aware of the massive confusion about alternative medicine that uncritical media coverage has often brought about. Outrageous claims are made for its apparent benefits, while at the same time well-proven, established, conventional medical practices are rubbished or dismissed.

Orthodox medicine is powerful. It can certainly save lives in critical situations, but in less acute circumstances it also has the ability to produce serious side effects, and it can create iatrogenic diseases, that is illnesses caused by doctors themselves (see page 41), and a complete disempowerment and passivity within patients. Alternative medicine, on the other hand, is gentler, and at the same time allows the patient much greater responsibility for his or her own health. It should never be considered for life-threatening situations such as meningitis, diabetes or appendicitis, but for the vast majority of ailments and symptoms experienced by people who wish to feel better, it offers a tremendous potential for physical, emotional and spiritual support. For the chronic diseases like rheumatoid arthritis and strokes, where traditional doctors all too often throw in the towel, alternative medicine is a crutch. For all those stress-related problems, such as migraine, palpitations and irritable bowel syndrome, it is a comfort. For those controversial disorders associated with our polluted modern environment, like ME (myalgic encephalomyelitis), attention deficit hyperactivity disorder, asthma and food intolerance, it is a tonic. For emotional and psychological difficulties, such as anxiety, depression and panic attacks, it is a godsend. For the large proportion of patients who see their doctor for non-specific or vague symptoms which do not fit into any neat or convenient category of recognized disease, it offers choice. To the thousands of people who, by dint of their lifestyles, have never realized their full potential for good health and fitness, it shows a new way forward. And finally, for all those who wish desperately to find some help with coming to terms with disability or even terminal illness whilst remaining in control of their own destiny, alternative medicine promises hope and preservation of the spirit.

Alternative medicine can therefore achieve many things. But there is also much it cannot achieve. It, too, has its limitations. Contrary to popular belief it is not always safe, natural, free of side effects and successful. Much of it is unregulated, its practitioners a law unto themselves and its benefits over-exaggerated and scientifically unproven. It also costs patients time and money. How can people make sense of it all? How do they decide which therapist they should take their symptoms to, and which of the various treatments would be appropriate for them? Never before has a full and proper answer to the question, 'Doctor, what's the alternative?' been so badly needed. This book, I hope, provides that answer.

PART ONE

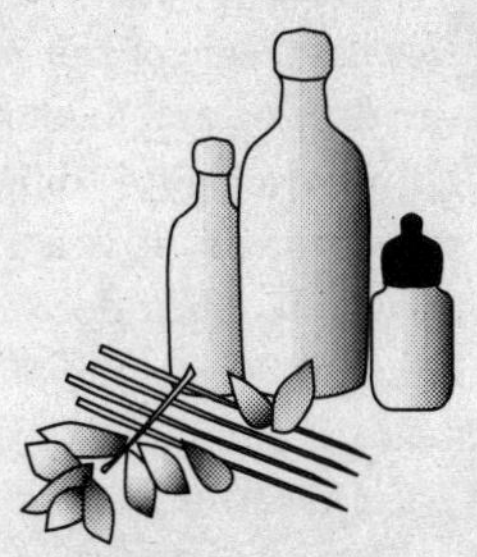

Complementary Versus Orthodox Medicine

[illegible] certain complementary therapies can be [illegible]. It is difficult [illegible] the [illegible] fully qualified and reputable [illegible] do you know you will not [illegible] taken for an expensive [illegible]. How will you cope with [illegible] of your doctor when he [illegible] out you have taken yourself off to see a 'charlatan' or [illegible] quack' and how will he react [illegible] undertake

CHAPTER 1

Complementary Therapy and You

The popularity of complementary therapy is increasing all the time, but even now only a small proportion of the population have actually tried it in any tangible form. Some people have had a bit of massage down at the health club; others have tried their grandmother's cure for sinusitis or arthritis, or have bought a little bottle of Rescue Remedy from the chemist or health shop when they were feeling particularly tense and edgy.

Growing numbers of people have become increasingly aware of the limitations of orthodox medical care and the side effects its treatment can bring on, and the mystique and promise of ancient Eastern medical philosophies is novel and attractive to many, but how likely would *you* be to use a complementary medicine? Perhaps a friend of yours has recommended it. Perhaps something you read has encouraged you to believe it might be the final answer to that chronic problem with which you have been perpetually plagued. Maybe you have become fed up with the paltry few minutes your GP can afford you each time you go to see him or her, or the hastily written but useless prescription automatically doled out to you. Possibly you are just disillusioned with the appliance of science to your complex and emotionally based difficulties, and wish to experiment with a more holistic and spiritual approach to these problems. You are held back, however, by niggling doubts. The cost of visiting certain complementary therapists can be substantial. It is difficult to ensure that the therapist you choose is fully qualified and reputable. How do you know you will not just be taken for an expensive ride? How will you cope with the wrath of your doctor when he finds out you have taken yourself off to see a 'charlatan' or a 'quack' and how will he react if you undertake alternative treatment without having been referred to the therapist by him? What will your friends think when they find out what you have done? Will they tease you? Laugh at you? Or might they be curious, intrigued, envious even?

In my 20 or so years of medical practice I have come to believe that certain people, certain personalities, are more naturally attracted to complementary therapies than others. Anyone can benefit from these treatments, however stoical, unemotional and sceptical they may be at the outset, but some patients, by dint of their upbringing, their outlook on life and their medical experiences, will always be more ready to embrace the generally less scientific and somewhat mystical system of health care known as complementary medicine.

To find out how likely *you* might be to experiment with and benefit from complementary therapy, I have devised a quiz which will give you at least a rough idea. Answer the questions in turn without pausing too long or thinking too hard about them, then count up your score at the end to discover how you relate to complementary medicine at this moment in time. When you have read the rest of this book, do the quiz again. You might be surprised to discover your outlook has changed.

Quiz:
Would Complementary Medicine Suit You?

Answer ALWAYS, SOMETIMES or NEVER to each of the following statements. The scoring system and what your score reveals about you is explained at the end.

1
- a You have symptoms that have been present for some time.
- b You have several apparently unrelated symptoms.
- c You have puzzling complaints which your doctor fails to recognize.
- d Your doctor tells you you have just got to live with your problems.
- e Your treatment fails to relieve your symptoms.

2
- a Your symptoms come and go.
- b You feel better when you are away on holiday.
- c You take regular vitamin or mineral supplements.
- d You try eliminating certain foodstuffs from your diet.
- e You are a vegetarian or a vegan.

3
- a You read the stars and take an interest in astrology.
- b You believe in ghosts
- c You believe aliens have visited Earth.
- d You have faith in God.
- e You find hospital treatment too impersonal.

4
- a You feel your doctor hardly knows you.
- b Visits to your doctor fail to reassure you.
- c A visit to your doctor upsets you.
- d A visit to your doctor leaves important things unsaid.
- e Your doctor is baffled by your problems.

5
- a Your doctor is awkward to talk to.
- b Your doctor makes you feel nervous or embarrassed.
- c Your doctor gives you pills or medications when you see him/her.
- d You are intrigued by miracle cures for illnesses.
- e You believe your personality strongly influences your health.

6
- a You believe your emotions strongly affect your health.
- b You drink alcohol in great moderation.
- c You are careful about what you eat.
- d You worry about your bowels.
- e You would attend a stress-management course if it were offered.

7
- a You believe anything natural is healthier.
- b You would be willing to pay for private treatment of your choice.
- c You worry about your health.
- d Your family is unlucky with their health.
- e You are unlikely to take what your doctor has prescribed for you.

8
- a Your doctor says there is nothing more he can do for you.
- b Most of your medical tests are normal.
- c Certain foods upset you.
- d You suffer from allergies.
- e You use a water filter or purifier at home.

9
- a You drink decaffeinated coffee.
- b You use detox diets.
- c You go on fasting diets for other than religious reasons.

d You worry about cancer.
e You worry about the use of antibiotics in modern farming.

10
a You believe ME (chronic fatigue syndrome) exists.
b You believe Gulf War syndrome exists.
c You are affected by environmental pollution.
d You feel tired all the time.
e You sleep well at night.

11
a You are a born worrier.
b You believe in spiritual healing.
c You are superstitious.
d You regard the pharmaceutical industry with suspicion.
e You wish your doctor would make you feel more important.

12
a Your doctor makes judgements about you.
b You wish your doctor was more on your wavelength.
c You experience troublesome side effects from your treatment.
d Despite having tests you still do not get a satisfactory diagnosis.
e You are keen to take steps now to prevent future illness.

13
a You regularly use health shops.
b You use essential oils and moisturizers.
c You believe in reincarnation.
d You are suspicious of and hostile to vaccination campaigns.
e The treatment of terminal illness frightens you.

14
- a You believe most illnesses could be prevented by changes in lifestyle.
- b You believe in the concept of a 'good death'.
- c You worry more than others about dying.
- d You avoid going to the doctor in case something serious is found.
- e You are dissatisfied with the service you get from your GP.

15
- a Your GP fails to take your problems seriously.
- b Your GP seems out of date and ill-informed.
- c You are concerned about the damage caused by passive smoking.
- d You are unhappy about putting yourself entirely in the hands of doctors.
- e You avoid over-the-counter remedies for minor ailments.

16
- a Asking your doctor for prescriptions is the last thing on your mind.
- b In your heart of hearts you feel neither your GP nor your specialist is really on your side.
- c You are more laid back than ambitious and competitive.
- d You are not bothered if your treatment has not been scientifically tried and tested first.
- e You are fascinated by accounts of out-of-body experiences.

THE SCORING SYSTEM

For every ALWAYS answer, score 3.
For every SOMETIMES answer, score 2.
For every NEVER answer, score 1.

Interpretation of Results

Score 80–120

You are generally quite satisfied with your GP and any hospital treatment you may have had. Your symptoms have always conformed to classical patterns of recognized illness and have responded to conventional treatment. You have a scientific approach to medical treatment, trust your advisers and are happy to be guided by them. You understand that invasive investigations and treatments are sometimes necessary to get to the root of the problem and make an accurate diagnosis, and you feel that new medical technology and pharmaceutical preparations are a godsend. You are highly unlikely to want to try complementary therapy in any shape or form and probably regard its practitioners with suspicion and amusement.

Score 121–200

On the whole you have kept an open mind about certain complementary therapies, although you still regard some of them as being rather 'wacky' and eccentric. You have been interested to hear about the experiences of some of your friends and colleagues who have tried alternative treatments with sometimes impressive results. Moreover, you do not always get the help you are looking for from your own doctor and have been frustrated at times by delays or poor service. If you were really sick and poorly you would always go to your GP first, but for minor, niggling things which your doctor does not seem too interested in, you might occasionally make an appointment with a complementary therapist. It is likely that in the future you will increasingly use complementary therapy in conjunction with traditional medical practices, and people with higher scores in this range will probably use both in roughly equal proportions.

Score 201–240

Complementary therapy will always be your first choice of

treatment since it encompasses all your ideals and philosophies regarding holistic health care. You are careful and particular about how you live your life. Your symptoms and problems are not the result of physical illness but are evidence of some spiritual or emotional malaise and you try to counterbalance as much of the devastation to nature that takes place around you as you can.

You are dissatisfied with orthodox medicine, you do not see eye to eye with your doctor, you hate hospitals and the impersonal care you receive there, and you feel that invasive procedures and powerful drugs produce just as much harm as good. You believe science in itself is not omniscient and omnipotent, and has often proved to be flawed. Complementary therapy, on the other hand, is safer, is less likely to produce iatrogenic disease (see page 41) and calls upon energies and influences which even the most modern scientific thinking cannot understand or explain. Complementary therapy employs gentle, natural methods which prevent illness in the first place by restoring harmony, balance and a fluent flow of energy within the body. The human body possesses the power to heal itself but modern medicine often obstructs this.

If your score is within this high range, you are someone who would have to be dragged, kicking and screaming, to a conventional doctor, and then only if you had a very acute or serious illness or had been advised to do so by your complementary practitioner.

CHAPTER 2

The Benefits of Orthodox Medicine

Orthodox Medicine, Past and Present

In view of the burgeoning popularity of alternative medicine, the number of therapists practising it and the amount of money spent by patients on acquiring its benefits, it would be easy to believe that conventional medicine had somehow failed us all. Yet this is clearly not the case. In fact, the complete opposite is true: modern twentieth-century medicine has dramatically revolutionized the health and welfare of the entire world, and its achievements should never be underestimated or belittled. That the planet's population has effectively doubled in the last 50 years bears testimony to this and provides ample evidence of the success that orthodox medicine has had in the struggle against overwhelming and life-threatening disease. Until recently, life expectancy was very much shorter than it is today and infant mortality was appalling. Every other baby born at the beginning of the century died before reaching the age of five, often from infectious diseases that we now consider trivial and harmless. In fact, so complacent have we now become that any death from infection of any kind comes as a considerable shock; every case of meningitis, for example, once a very common cause of death in the general population, is now headline news. To a large extent it is precisely because of the achievements of twentieth-century orthodox medicine that a resurgence in interest in complementary therapies has been allowed to take place. In many ways it is a luxury engendered by a population made increasingly healthy by decades of successful conventional health care which has conquered many grave diseases and provided enormous relief for all those who would otherwise have suffered.

A Brief History of Orthodox Medicine

In the earliest culture, any form of doctoring or healing was usually associated with religion. Ill-health and disease were generally regarded as a punishment from some divine deity or spirit, and much of the treatment on offer was directed at purging the evil within and exorcising malevolent influences. The oldest evidence of surgical procedures carried out for these purposes comes in the firm evidence of refined skulls dating back some 10,000 years. Sharpened stone tools were used to bore holes in the patient's skull in the hope of letting out the evil spirits that were producing the symptoms of insanity, epilepsy or uncontrolled aggression for which the patient was being treated. But the technicians performing such procedures were more like priests than physicians, and it was not until the fifth century BC, at the time of Hippocrates, that medicine itself was established as a recognized profession.

Hippocrates was the real father of modern medicine as we know it, establishing a sound body of knowledge and a code of ethics which was then passed on to each generation of medical men and women. In fact, these firm ethical principles, as laid down in the Hippocratic oath, are still used to this day as a guide to doctors, although the oath is no longer formally sworn and witnessed, but merely agreed to in the spirit of tradition. After the magnificent contribution of Hippocrates, and his emphasis on the holistic approach to healing and the scientific evaluation of treatment, the world had to wait an inordinately long time for medicine to progress further. Several centuries passed before the advent of the Renaissance when change suddenly began to take place.

The Age of Discovery

In 1543, Andreas Vesalius produced the first accurate anatomical work. In the seventeenth century William Harvey demonstrated how blood circulates through the body, and Antonj Vanleeuwenhoek identified micro-organisms and cellular structures with the help of the light microscope, which he himself had developed. Late in the following century, Edward Jenner amazed his colleagues and co-workers by developing the principle of vaccination. But it was not until the nineteenth century that modern medicine became truly scientific in its overall approach and based itself on rigidly systematic observation, analysis and experimentation. Louis Pasteur's work on the germ theory of disease contributed hugely to the understanding of illness transmission and the prevention and containment of epidemics.

The Age of Invention

New inventions, such as the medical thermometer, the stethoscope and the ophthalmoscope, pushed the frontiers of knowledge further. The first X-rays of the body were taken in 1895 by Wilhelm Roentgen, and just 10 years later clear radiological evidence of kidney function was made possible by the use of radio-opaque X-ray contrast medium. Early in the twentieth century, physicians began to make more dramatic inroads into the provision of effective treatments. Cholera, diphtheria and typhoid, diseases that had accounted for countless thousands of deaths in previous years, were now preventable by vaccination, and improved sanitation seriously reduced the threat from these diseases. General anaesthesia, first demonstrated by the American surgeon Crawford Long in 1842 using ether, became safer and more effective and, coupled with Joseph Lister's antiseptic surgical techniques, made the result of operative procedures very much more acceptable.

The Pharmaceutical Revolution

At the beginning of the Second World War, penicillin was still being developed in the laboratory, and remained rationed, largely for use by servicemen, throughout the conflict. After the war its widespread use dramatically reduced mortality from hitherto common infections, such as pneumonia, septicaemia, osteomyelitis and meningitis, and undoubtedly saved millions upon millions of lives. Even tuberculosis, probably the oldest single most important cause of death in the developed world, was all but vanquished with the advent of BCG vaccination and the development of the antibiotic streptomycin.

Thereafter, newer and more sophisticated drugs appeared and the pharmacological revolution proceeded apace. Insulin was available in a variety of forms for people with diabetes who, before 1940, would have died soon after diagnosis. Patients with deficiency diseases could now be cured quickly, and psychotropic medication, such as chlorpromazine, made a huge difference to the management of sufferers of mental illness. Cortisone proved yet another dramatic life-saver across the board, and enabled surgeons to crack on with their increasingly impressive programme of organ transplantation without the worry of otherwise inevitable organ graft rejection. In the 1950s, the oral contraceptive pill was developed, something which arguably did more in practical terms to emancipate women than the whole of the suffragette movement put together.

Towards a Medical Utopia?

In the 1940s and 1950s, surgical cardiology forged ahead, offering 'blue babies' with congenital heart disease the chance of life, and adults with coronary heart disease the possibility of open heart surgery or a coronary bypass operation. In 1967, Christian Barnard made history when he transplanted a woman's heart into the chest of Louis Washkansky. He lived for 18 days. Today, heart transplant operations are commonplace and no longer groundbreaking, with at least two thirds of patients surviving five years or more. During all this time other exciting scientific advances promised the prospect of an almost unimaginable medical utopia: the deaf were fitted with miniature electric hearing aids, and the poorly sighted were able to replace their glasses with contact lenses; kidney stones could be shattered from outside the body without even touching the patient, courtesy of shock-wave lithotripsy; and in 1978 the world's first 'test-tube baby', Louise Brown, was born in England as a result of in vitro fertilization techniques; better investigative and diagnostic methods using cardiac catheterization, fibre-optic endoscopes, scanners and monoclonal antibodies have helped pinpoint medical abnormalities more easily and accurately; chorionic villus sampling even allows the detection of genetic disorders in an unborn and developing foetus of just eight weeks' gestation.

Indeed, it sometimes seems that, today, mainstream medicine can achieve almost anything: bone marrow transplantation can offer a final chance of a cure to patients with leukaemia in whom chemotherapy has failed to bring about a remission; surgeons can operate on babies whilst they are still in the womb; organs and tissues can be excised through tiny key hole incisions; lasers can obliterate damaged blood vessels at the back of the eye to prevent blindness; and infertile couples can be granted the miracle of medically assisted conception.

Recent Progress in Therapeutics

The pharmaceutical industry, too can boast impressive continued success and can feel justifiably proud. State of the art treatments for a wide range of conditions, from AIDS to heart disease are major advances where previously there was little or no hope of long-term survival. Millions of people affected by conditions like diabetes, schizophrenia, ulcers and cancer, have been able to resume a working life thanks to effective drug treatments. It is not only the patients themselves who have appreciated these advances, but their families, carers and friends, too, all of whom are otherwise touched by the patients' continued suffering. Many of these newer drugs have reduced or eliminated the need for other more costly treatments. For example, over the last 40 years, prescription drugs have enabled the number of hospital admissions in 12 major disease areas to be halved, and modern anaesthetics have allowed day surgery to be relied on much more heavily, thereby freeing other resources in the NHS for treating patients more rapidly and cheaply. The country's economy is also boosted as the cost of ill-health is reduced. In Britain, in 1997, 187 million working days were lost through sickness at a direct cost to employers of 12 billion pounds, so any savings in this made possible by modern drugs are a very positive contribution.

Having all but eliminated the scourge of acute infectious diseases in our society, the pharmaceutical industry has concentrated in recent years on improving the quality of life. Consider, for example, the value of medicines in the treatment of epilepsy, asthma and breast cancer. More than 300,000 people in Britain are affected by epilepsy, more than 80 per cent of whom have their seizures controlled with the minimum of side effects courtesy of modern anticonvulsants. More than 3 million people in Britain are diagnosed with asthma, 1.3 million of whom are children. The annual mortality from this condition is somewhere in the region of 1,600, but it appears to be dropping by about 6 per cent per year due to an improved understanding of the disease, the setting up of consensus guidelines on the management of asthma, and, last but by no means least, the increased prescribing of appropriate drugs. Nearly 35,000 women every year are newly diagnosed as having breast cancer, and the annual mortality rate is 14,000. As the number of new diagnoses exceeds the death rate, it is calculated that around 105,000 women are living with breast cancer in Britain at any one time. Despite very slow progress in the overall rate of cure for breast cancer, chemotherapy has without doubt brought about better outcomes for the disease. Average annual survival rates have increased by 16 per cent and the average recurrence rate has dropped by more than a quarter with particularly good results amongst younger women. The development of anti-cancer medicines for previously untreatable advanced breast cancer has also offered the chance of further extended and better quality life. Great work is also going on in other fields, notably those of coronary artery disease, HIV and AIDS, depression and peptic ulcers, yet despite these achievements there still remain frontiers to penetrate and breakthroughs to make. Drug-resistant tuberculosis and malaria are both becoming more prevalent, with 300 million affected by the latter worldwide, 2 million of whom will perish every year.

New Challenges

As fewer people are dying prematurely from other conditions due to the benefits bestowed by insulin, antibiotics and beta-blockers, proportionately greater numbers of people are developing and dying from cancer. Out of any 60 people, 20 will be diagnosed with cancer at some point in their lives and 15 will die from it. Cancer is now second only to heart disease as the biggest killer in Britain, and 1 million people in the country currently suffer from it.

The effective treatment of cancer is, however, just one of the many challenges facing the future of modern medical practice. Viral infections, including AIDS, are another challenging area, along with congenital and hereditary disease. In the next decade, gene therapy might make it possible to introduce undamaged copies of a defective gene into a patient's body so that a single fault responsible for his or her symptoms may be overcome. If so, cystic fibrosis sufferers might be able to lead normal lives, patients with muscular dystrophy might be able to avoid disability, and haemophiliacs might never need another blood transfusion. The Human Genome project currently in operation aims to identify all the 100,000 or so individual genes which govern the functions of the human body. Since each gene is composed of twin-stranded DNA (deoxyribonucleic acid), this involves the intricate dissection of up to 3,000 million DNA base pairs in order to fulfil that goal.

Immunotherapy is another highly promising therapeutic possibility, based on the premise that monoclonal antibodies are specific to certain antigens – locking on to them and neutralizing them. An antigen is any substance that can trigger an immune response, resulting in the formation of antibodies designed to combat infection and disease. Since monoclonal antibodies can be cultivated in unlimited numbers in a laboratory, it might be possible to specifically target, say, cancer cells or arthritis-inducing inflammatory cells in the hope of destroying them, whilst leaving all other healthy tissues intact. Most existing therapies fail to do this, producing side effects and complications as a result.

Clinical Trials and Evidence-Based Medicine

Quite apart from the magnificent contribution to clinical medicine made in the last 100 years, orthodox medical practice has established a sound and often irrefutable scientific foundation to support and justify its methods and practices. Ever since the 1940s, randomized medical trials have been employed to demonstrate scientifically and accurately whether any new drug, treatment or surgical intervention of any kind is effective, safe and superior to or at least as good as any existing therapies. These trials also reveal any effect or adverse reaction caused by the treatment that might not have been suspected from experimentation on animals.

Randomized clinical trials are very carefully set up expressly to eliminate any misleading results. Personal bias and the placebo effect (where a person's expectations of the treatment alter the way the person perceives the effect) must be ruled out if the trial is to be of any true value, and the randomized trial effectively achieves just that. Certainly no better or more reliable method of evaluation has ever been described. By the time the results have also been subjected to rigorous and repeated statistical analysis, scientists are generally prepared to believe the treatment really does work because the results and observations witnessed are repeatable and verifiable by other researchers; the consistency and reliability of the results can be tested and proved.

Any good trial is designed in such a way as to subject the treatment to the test of refutability. That is to say that before a hypothesis or assumption can be accepted, research has to try extremely hard to disprove it, but must ultimately fail to do so. It sounds complicated (the design of this model of trial is described as 'hypothetico-deductive') but experts agree that it is the only real test of credible, irrefutable fact. The use of any alternative method might result in a false claim that given treatment can work in every single case – an incorrect and potentially dangerous state of affairs. But not only is the randomized clinical trial reliable; it has also been invaluable for detecting which treatments are best for patients. It has shown the medical profession how best to treat those with breast cancer or leukaemia, whether one drug is better than another and whether symptoms of a disease are a side effect of the treatment or a complication of the disease itself.

One of the problems with the randomized clinical trial, however, is that although meaningful results are relatively easy to achieve if the disease being treated is a serious and significant one, it is much harder to obtain definite results when the illness is milder, less concrete or subject to any degree of controversy. For example, the benefits of intravenous benzylpenicillin in the treatment of meningitis septicaemia are plain to see, but it is much harder to prove that nutritional manipulation helps a patient suffering from chronic arthritis. Similarly, scientific results are not so easy to interpret when an ailment is less serious or its symptoms less significant and vague. In such cases, it is much more difficult to establish that any improvement in the patient's condition can indeed be attributed to the treatment and could not have happened purely by chance. By contrast, amongst the many difficulties encountered in trying to make many complementary therapies more scientific and acceptable is that many such treatments do not lend themselves at all easily to the concept of the randomized clinical trial and the hypothetico deductive model.

Professional Training

There are further extraordinary strengths of which conventional medicine can rightly be proud. The education of its students and practitioners is organized, defined and extremely rigorous, and, in general, it is only fully qualified doctors who have contact with patients. Furthermore, its governing body, the General Medical

Council (GMC) insists on a professional code of conduct and ethics as well as disciplinary procedures for all doctors in the event of any medical misdemeanours. The duties of all doctors registered with the GMC are clearly established and set out in the GMC's booklet 'Good Medical Practice'. This states that patients must be able to trust doctors with their lives and well-being. It states that to justify that trust, the medical profession has a duty to maintain a good standard of practice and care, and to show respect for human life. It goes on to say that above all doctors must:

- Make the care of the patient their first concern.
- Treat every patient politely and considerately.
- Respect the patient's dignity and privacy.
- Listen to patients and respect their views.
- Give patients information in a way they can understand.
- Respect the rights of patients to be fully involved in decisions about their care.
- Keep professional knowledge and skills up to date.
- Recognize the limits of their professional competence.
- Be honest and trustworthy.
- Respect and protect confidential information.
- Make sure that their personal beliefs do not prejudice their patients' care.
- Act quickly to protect patients from risk if there is good reason to believe that they or a colleague may not be fit to practise.
- Avoid abusing their position as a doctor.
- Work with colleagues in ways that best serve patients' interests.

If all complementary therapies could mirror such careful regulation of its practices, many more would be readily accepted by the orthodox medical establishment. Until that happens, alternative medicine will continue to be regarded with suspicion and antagonism by many within the profession. Outside the profession, however, the lack of scientific justification for many complementary therapies does not seem to bother people. In fact, the authoritarian image of traditional doctors, with their stuffy academic and somewhat supercilious approach to patients and their problems, is the main reason why many are eschewing what twentieth-century mainstream medicine has to offer.

Changing Expectations

Ironically, despite the considerable triumphs and dramatic breakthroughs in the evolution of modern medicine, a growing number of people are coming to regard conventional medical practice with increasing scepticism and intolerance. How can this be? Our population owes a huge debt of gratitude to the pioneers and researchers who devoted their lives to bringing about the miracles of modern health care; many people would not even be alive today but for their ground-breaking efforts. But evidence of the growing dissatisfaction and disillusionment with orthodox medicine is unmistakable. It seems clear that science alone is not enough to satisfy all the needs of today's patients, and that it is simply too stark and powerful in its current undiluted form. When patients consult doctors, they are seeking something more than that which can be provided by dispensing a prescription or performing an operation. The doctor–patient relationship has been eroded and weakened by a number of factors, and patients' expectations have altered beyond recognition over the last two or three decades. The euphoria of the medical utopia of the 1940s onwards has been followed by much more widespread awareness of the limitations of modern medicine.

CHAPTER 3

The Limitations of Orthodox Medicine

The Clinical Picture

The brave new medical world anticipated during the middle part of the twentieth century has not been realized. The pandemic of AIDS has forced many to reconsider the threat from infectious disease, and increased longevity has left many apprehensive about degenerative diseases, heart disease and cancer. The outlook for patients with Alzheimer's disease and schizophrenia is of huge concern to those families whose lives are touched by the consequences, and only very slow progress has been made by medical researchers in preventing or treating these conditions. Care of the chronically or terminally ill leaves many patients feeling unsupported and without hope, and sufferers of poly-symptomatic but nebulous complaints such as ME (myalgic encephalomyelitis) or irritable bowel syndrome feel hopelessly let down by conventional doctors because so many physicians are dismissive and judgemental when faced with symptoms that science itself struggles to explain.

The art and science of diagnosis still remains the speciality of orthodox doctors but, even now, many symptoms elude identification and categorization, leaving patients with very real problems to face when the implication is that they are not really ill or in need of help. Many diseases still defy diagnosis despite the vast array of expensive and sophisticated technological equipment available to doctors, and lives are still lost to cancer where the primary source of the tumour has yet to be identified. Doctors find it increasingly difficult to keep up to date with the rapid changes in therapeutic practices and guidelines. Moreover, new technology originally intended to make life easier for the medical profession has in fact increased work and stress levels, and merely confused and distracted doctors as much as it has benefited them. Consequently, many are still uncertain whether they believe that newly described conditions, such as attention deficit hyperactivity disorder, dyslexia, food intolerance, seasonal affective disorder, chronic fatigue syndrome and Gulf War syndrome, are genuine diseases or not. There cannot be much hope for patients suffering from any of these conditions if the doctors they are consulting do not even know whether they exist or not! For too long doctors have been programmed to believe that if the patient does not at first respond to their therapeutic endeavours, then they are not really ill, oblivious to the fact that fear and anxiety about illness are factors which in themselves need addressing.

The Limitations of the System

The British National Health Service may still be regarded in some respects as the envy of the world, but there is much about it that severely limits the ability of doctors to satisfy all the needs of their patients. In general practice, the average size of a family doctor's list is 2,200 patients, for all of whom he or she might be responsible from the cradle to the grave. Bizarrely, since the family doctor is paid per capita, the more patients he has on his list, the more income he receives, despite the fact that the more patients he sees, the less time he has available to spend with each one. In effect, the doctor becomes richer while his patients' health care becomes poorer. This system obviously discourages better working practices. The six minutes per patient for the average consultation is woefully inadequate, including, as it must, time for a full history to be obtained, for the patient to undress, for a full physical examination to be made, and for the development of an investigation plan followed by discussion of any appropriate treatment and follow-up. Most doctors find it difficult to find out much about their patients' lifestyles, their expectations, their fears and their anxieties within this consultation framework, and most patients find it impossible to voice their anxieties and apprehensions or put across the exact nature of their problems or symptoms in the time available. It is a system that is disease orientated rather than health orientated, based as it is on the patient attending the doctor's surgery once problems have already developed. This is, of course, changing gradually with the establishment of 'well woman' and 'well man' screening clinics, and other 'health promotion activities' for patients suffering from given disorders such as asthma and diabetes, but for far too many people the doctor's surgery is still seen as a place to go when you are ill, rather than a healing centre from which to obtain advice on staying fit and healthy in the future.

For most patients requiring help, the GP's surgery is the first port of call, and the family doctor is seen as a sort of overall gatekeeper for patients with illnesses requiring treatment under the NHS. It is he or she who decides which patients are referred to specialist hospital clinics and how urgently this takes place. Although NHS treatment is free of charge at the point of delivery, this state-run system has two distinct disadvantages. Firstly, it deprives the patients of the value of paying for their treatment directly. In many other countries and in other health systems, the financial transaction between the patient and the therapist is direct. The patient actually hands money to the doctor when the consultation or treatment take place. This may be a psychological advantage in that it frees the patient from any suspicion of state rationing of health provision, and helps make both the doctor and the patient aware, as it were, of what they are getting. Defenders of the NHS would argue that this system disadvantages the poor and the most needy, but it is nevertheless the type of system employed for the most part by alternative medical practitioners practising complementary therapy, and may well be one of the many reasons for its success and popularity. Put simply, there is a lot to be said for knowing that you are getting what you pay for.

The second disadvantage of the 'free' state-run GP system system is that it results in NHS family doctors spending probably

80 per cent of their time with 20 per cent of their patients, not because they are the most needy, but because there is no disincentive to stop them occupying this much of the doctor's time; if patients had to pay each time they saw their doctor, they would visit only when really necessary.

The hospital system also has its critics. Waiting lists are ridiculously long in some instances; patients with coronary heart disease, for example, are sometimes expected to wait up to a year and a half for treatment, even under the terms of the official Patient's Charter. Many others requiring hip replacement, cataract surgery or hysterectomy are having to wait inordinately long periods of time, and even those with potentially malignant breast lumps and suspicious changes of bowel habit suggestive of bowel tumours are unable to see specialists adequately urgently. The current system leaves patients fed up at having to see a different doctor every time they visit a clinic, and there is increasing intolerance when clinical records are mislaid or lost and when communication continually breaks down. Patients become confused when they are sent from one specialist to the next without adequate explanation or rationale, and although they understand why medical and nursing staff may be demoralized, they see themselves as the ultimate victims of this.

It seems there is little the patient can do to escape this disintegrating system of conventional health care. One large supermarket chain, stimulated by what they perceived as an increased interest in self-screening amongst their customers, introduced self-testing urine strips to detect undiagnosed diabetes. The British Medical Association (BMA) criticized their campaign on the basis that it would alarm people unnecessarily. However, if the medical profession acknowledges that for every one of the 1.4 million people in Britain with diabetes there is another who is not yet diagnosed, the BMA must also acknowledge that the profession is failing to identify these vulnerable people. The general population are obviously increasingly interested in taking responsibility for their own health, and there is a great deal to commend this. In fact, since the urine strips were introduced further do-it-yourself screening kits have been made available for sale to the public with considerable commercial success. Consumers have long had access to home pregnancy and ovulation tests, but they can now also screen themselves for a dozen separate conditions using the urine test strips, and they can identify the presence of blood in their stools and high cholesterol levels in their circulation.

The Training and Attitude of Our Doctors

Conventional medical training is disease centred, so it has become easy for some doctors to come to regard patients merely as walking illnesses rather than people. Casualty officers are often guilty of referring to 'the appendix in cubicle three' or 'the head injury in Resuscitation', and are more enthusiastic about the fact that a particular patient is 'an interesting case' than that they are in dire need of caring and sympathetic treatment. It seems that doctors' training, focused as it is on biochemistry, physiology and anatomy, and then reinforced with pharmacology, medical physics and chemical pathology, has made them rather distant and inhumane. They have lost many of the interpersonal skills which their predecessors once held in abundance, and they are no longer very good at the art of doctoring in itself. Up to 50 per cent of illness is psycho-social or emotional in origin, so doctors today are, in fact, trained to deal with only a small proportion of the problems they see in medical practice. When a patient has non-specific, low-grade and nebulous symptoms which do not fall neatly into any easily recognized pattern of disease, doctors fall back on esoteric diagnostic tests in the hope of identifying the malady. They forget that some people feel ill even when there is no disease process responsible, and that other patients may feel very well, whilst simultaneously harbouring some progressive condition. Moreover, today's doctors seem unwilling to listen to what the patient is actually telling them, to such a degree that 'What seems to be the trouble?' (with the emphasis on '*seems*') has become a modern medical catchphrase, implying that the doctor has little interest in what the patient believes is the trouble, because ultimately only the doctor is in any position to decide.

There is other evidence that doctors do not listen effectively to their patients and that many are so wrapped up and obsessed with the technology available that the beliefs, fears and expectations of their patients are ignored. There was a time when patients were highly impressed by sophisticated tests, and the more invasive the investigations they received were, the luckier they felt themselves to be. This has now turned full circle, and there is a growing feeling that over-investigation and excessively aggressive treatment can in itself cause damage. Many a stroke has been caused by passing catheters into furred up, hardened carotid arteries, and many a hollow organ of the abdomen has been perforated as a result of unnecessary invasive diagnostic techniques. Such cases are now so common that, these days, part of the GP's role has become not only to diagnose patients appropriately, and to refer them for treatment, but also to protect them from over-investigation at the hands of specialists looking to extend their own medical prowess and enhance their own academic reputations. Many medical investigations are carried out purely to protect doctors from the possibility of litigation. As the number of claims of malpractice by doctors continues to rise in parallel with what has been happening in the United States for the last decade or two, the need to cover every possible diagnostic eventuality, and so subject patients to a barrage of tests, overwhelms the system as well as the sensibilities of the patient. In this way the patient is further removed from the magic and charisma of the individual therapist, and will find waiting for the cold clinical results a thoroughly depersonalizing experience.

The Placebo Effect

The system under which conventional doctors are trained is so rigidly controlled by the dictates of science that it fails to allow any possibility for the mystical and supernatural side of healing which so many patients obviously need. Any useful effect derived from any kind of treatment that is not directly due to the treatment itself acting on the disease, or on the patient, is called the 'placebo effect'. The 'placebo' is the treatment – be it a chemically inert drug, a physical treatment or even a spiritual experience – which brings this about.

Placebos are liberally and universally used by complementary therapists, and even the most hardened academic professors acknowledge that at least 30 per cent of the benefit a patient gains from the treatment is the result of the placebo effect. However, they are never prescribed by orthodox doctors on the basis that they are unscientific; in fact the prescription of any placebo in clinical medical practice in the UK is expressly forbidden by the GMC. This brutally ethical, honest and, some would say, excessively purist approach deprives doctors of an invaluable tool, and is mistaken by many a patient as a sign that the doctor does not care or has nothing to offer. The training and attitudes of our modern-day doctors leave much to be desired.

Forgotten Skills

In theory, a century of steady diagnostic progress, increasingly sharpened clinical skills and sophisticated treatments should have produced knowledgeable, dedicated, vocationally trained specialists whose medical acumen was second to none. In practice, however, such a variety of diagnostic technology has led to clinical confusion and economic rationing which has rendered much of it unavailable to or inappropriate for many patients, and physical examination skills have plummeted with increased emphasis on laboratory tests, scans and X-rays. The simple skill of taking a history from a patient is nowhere near as detailed and all-encompassing as it used to be. Celebrated educators used to remind yesterday's medical students that 90 per cent of diagnoses could be made simply by listening to the patient's description of his or her symptoms. Listen, they exhorted, and the patient will tell you the diagnosis. But history-taking today is cursory and assumptive; the first problem identified tends to be the one quickly homed in on, the doctor acting like a medical Exocet reaching the first identifiable object in its path. The plethora of different treatments available for most medical conditions also gives a real and lasting impression of indecision and dithering to those on the receiving end, and the doctors who are faced with solving such therapeutic dilemmas often resort to the remedy with which they are most familiar (quite reasonably, for purposes of safety), rather than embarking on a new and possibly even more effective and better-tolerated alternative.

Plummeting Morale

As for dedication and vocational training, the morale and enthusiasm among Britain's family and hospital doctors is at an all-time low. Increasing workloads, expanding patient expectations, reduced resources, pressure on time, increasing litigation, rising professional indemnity costs and income held down to levels lower than inflation by successive governments have all promoted a general disillusionment and dissatisfaction with medical practice in Britain. More medical graduates are abandoning their careers within a year or two of qualifying than at any previous time, whilst the clamour to take early retirement at the other end of the chronological spectrum has never been greater. Few doctors wish to practise in inner-city locations, and more and more physicians, who set out on careers in medicine with hope, enthusiasm and good intention continue to practise their chosen specialities reluctantly regarding the privilege as more of a pain than a pleasure. Nor can many doctors hope to work in the field in which they are most interested. The queues for the top positions in the specialities of their choice grow ever longer, and many live with resentment at having to practise in a second-rate speciality in a third-rate location on fourth-rate pay.

Contrast this with the sunny dispositions of complementary therapists who work only in their chosen field, adopting and incorporating new ideas and practices as they wish. They can choose their own clientele, set up shop wherever they want, and remain free, by and large, of restrictions and limitations. They are financially rewarded according to how much they do and how good they are at what they do, much less likely to be sued, and may not even need to possess any experience or qualifications. Little wonder then, that the number of complementary therapists working in our society is increasing fast.

Gaps in Medical Knowledge

While complementary therapists may find their work more satisfying, their training is nowhere near as academic. Unlike these happier, less-regulated free agents, conventional doctors can at least boast a thorough educational grounding in biochemistry, anatomy and physiology. In the course of their six-to-seven-year training, they undoubtedly learn exactly how the body works and functions. In rotation, they spend time in each of the major medical disciplines, which, amongst other things, incorporates physical medicine, surgery, obstetrics and gynaecology, and psychiatry. They also cram in enormous amounts of pharmacological information while at the same time learning about difficult, delicate and sometimes dangerous invasive techniques such as cardiac catheterization, lumbar puncture and bronchial endoscopy. But even after these admittedly arduous years spent at medical school and the draconian and physically and mentally more exhausting post-graduate years, our contemporary doctors still remain woefully underprepared for the job our society expects them to carry out.

Thirty per cent of all consultations with the GP are for emotionally based or psychosocial problems, and a further 20 per cent relate to lifestyle issues or difficulties arising from something as simple as poor diet, yet modern medical students receive hardly any grounding in sex education, psychosexual counselling, emotional difficulties or clinical nutrition. Moreover, medical students tend to emanate from rather narrow middle-class backgrounds, and are largely deprived, by dint of their rigorous training, of very much experience of the 'real' world.

Their relative inexperience of life and its hassles is often horribly exposed. When it is, their instinct to fall back on organic and physical modules of disease processes often gets the better of them, and their defensive manner in the consultation room is easily misread as arrogant or judgemental (and sometimes arrogant or judgemental is exactly what they are!).

Physician Heal Thyself

In the course of their studies, medical students are also at risk of taking part in stereotypical social behaviour which might well shock or even horrify their future patients. Potentially dangerous pranks, alcoholic binges, experimentation with anaesthetic gases and heavy smoking all seem, in some circles at least, to be regarded as typical behaviour for medical students. I am happy to admit that my knowledge of this is based on careful observation of my own fellow-students, and that I have a modicum of personal experience in this area myself! Yet the black-humour-laden and cavalier approach to life so reminiscent of the famous TV series *MASH*, and so determinedly clung to by some doctors once they have qualified, is not popular with patients: they wonder why so many doctors insist that they change their diet when they are grossly overweight themselves; they are curious to know why some doctors still smoke; they cannot imagine their doctor ever exercising; they think it an ironic joke that while doctors frequently tell patients to reduce their levels of stress, they themselves are continually running late, have too many patients to deal with and far too little time in which to deal with them, and have one of the highest rates of alcoholism, divorce and suicide of any occupation. Patients are often left to puzzle over these discrepancies. Why is it that doctors do not practise what they preach? Why is there one rule for patients and another for doctors? It is almost as if doctors do not really believe what they are telling their patients; as if they do not care. The sad truth is that the vast majority of conventional doctors patently *do* care and apply a higher level of conscientiousness to their profession than many. It is just that they seem to have lost many of the qualities of the charismatic healer.

Doctors as Healers

Hippocrates, the father of modern medicine espoused a truly holistic philosophy of clinical practice which incorporated the physical appraisal of the patient's entire being. It never contrived to separate mind, body and soul, but expressly sought to treat them as a single confluent entity. Hippocrates was a charismatic healer. The fictitious doctors Cameron and Finlay of TV fame, practising in their native Tannochbrae some 60 years ago, looked after patients literally from the womb to the tomb, becoming in the process not just trusted physicians but friends, social workers, confidants, counsellors, priests and general pillars of society. These doctors, too, were charismatic healers.

One reason for the holistic attitude of such healers, however, was that medical science had very much less to offer at the time. Without penicillin or a cure for tuberculosis, and when poverty and poor sanitation and living standards abounded, they had no option but to try to make up for what was not yet available therapeutically with caring and charisma alone. The advent of powerful drugs, sophisticated diagnostic techniques, and a growing but naive public confidence that modern medicine could cure almost anything, gradually changed all that. Doctors became better equipped and achieved a superior cure rate in the treatment of severe disorders, but they simultaneously became more scientific, less charismatic and more remote. As far as those patients with more nebulous and non-specific symptoms were concerned, if their problems and difficulties failed to be explicable by innovative state of the art methods, the doctor did not believe they were ill at all. Such patients were often dismissed as neurotics, hypochondriacs or, even worse, hysterics.

Diagnosis and treatment became more remote, too. At one time, most doctors fully examined their patients, listening to their chest, palpating their abdominal organs and manipulating their spine and limbs, but this fairly intimate physical contact was replaced by the blood test, the X-ray and the urine analysis. Even the few remaining hands-on procedures, like postural drainage for chest infections and soothing massage for musculo-skeletal disorders, were carried out not by doctors themselves but by physiotherapists who simply followed the orders of the clinician in charge. The latter never seemed to want to get his hands 'dirty' any more. Even when he had to, it was only when protected by latex surgical gloves and a starched white coat. Regrettably, many of today's orthodox doctors seem devoid of the instinctive qualities of caring and healing that are so characteristic of their counterparts in complementary therapy (see Table 1).

TABLE 1:
Contrasting Consultation Styles in Conventional and Complementary Medicine

Feature	Orthodox	Complementary
Time	Average consultation time 6 mins per patient. Doctor is usually busy and hurried.	Average first consultation over 60 mins; 30 mins for follow-ups. Therapist attentive and unrushed.
Working environment	Stark. Institutionalized. Depersonalized.	Warm. Comfortable. Individual.
Listening ability	Poor. Doctor often interrupts. Hears only 'sound bites'. Often disagrees with patient's interpretation of symptoms.	Good attention to detail. Patient and thoughtful attention to client.
Treating patients as individuals	Doctor treats 'diseases' rather than personalities. Attempts to get all patients to conform to single neat category of illness.	Therapist sees the personality as crucial to the symptoms and the treatment.

Feature	Orthodox	Complementary
Dealing with emotions	Doctor often lacks empathy and sensitivity. Trained to be scientifically objective.	Practitioners are often gifted at expressing feelings and sympathy. Subjectivity deemed acceptable.
Continuity of care	Same doctor rarely seen twice for same ailment.	Patient will usually see same therapist.
Lifestyle considerations	Lifestyle, domestic and occupational factors rarely considered.	Lifestyle and social adjustments central to therapy.
Setting an example	Doctors often overweight or unfit; high rates of alcoholism, divorce and suicide.	Most practitioners are prime examples of what they preach.
Explaining	Not always good at keeping the patient fully informed.	Generally takes trouble to increase patient understanding.
Use of jargon	Automatic reversion to medical technology.	Pseudoscientific jargon creeping in but mostly simple and symbolic language.
Decisiveness	Plethora of diagnostic and treatment options often make doctor appear uncertain.	Expression of confidence and certainty in treatment selection.
Expressing the patient's chances	Legally responsible to be brutally honest, but truth often statistically complicated.	Optimism and positive thinking is paramount; anecdotal rather than statistical optimism.
Offering hope and encouragement	Often a neglected area. Running out of therapeutic options can lead to hopelessness and despair in the mentally ill.	Forms a major component of complementary healing.

Doctors and Compassion

If, as seems the case, precise diagnosis is not always possible, sympathy and caring are. Ask most patients what they would rather choose – a doctor who is friendly and approachable, explains everything to them and appears sympathetic, or an extremely well-qualified professor who may have a better understanding of the problem but who barks at the patient, as if 'casting pearls before swine', with scant regard for their sensitivity or feelings – and almost all will opt for the former. Most patients still prefer the carer to the consultant, and would choose the reliable family doctor, like Dr Cameron of *Dr Finlay's Casebook*, to the gung-ho surgeon Sir Lancelot Spratt of *Doctor in the House* fame. Both might be excellent in their individual fields but, as far as the patient is concerned, it is a matter of confidence and trust. It is partly because so many doctors who trained at the Sir Lancelot Spratt school of surgery are still practisng in this high-handed manner that so many infirm people prefer to stay from away from hospitals altogether. Instead of being regarded as centres of healing, where sick people go to recuperate and become well again, they are seen as depersonalizing hell holes where dreadful mistakes may occur, and where patients are treated as guinea-pigs or pin-cushions with no say whatsoever in the handling of their clinical care. In many London teaching hospitals, Sir Lancelot's tradition of ward rounds lives on even now. The consultants and their fawning medical teams surround the foot of the patient's bed and discuss their 'case' in detail without even so much as a proper, 'Hello. What's your name and how are you feeling?' Even worse, far from helping the patient to begin to understand his or her condition and explaining what the intention is with regard to its treatment, the medical team sometimes gives the impression of deliberately ensuring the patient *cannot* understand what is being said.

Medical Jargon

Another alienating penchant of the orthodox profession is the use of esoteric terminology based on Latin and Greek derivations ('jargon', in other words). This is hardly helpful when doctors are talking to and explaining matters to their patients. It deprives patients of any real comprehension or insight into their illness, and undoubtedly operates as a means of keeping the balance of power in the doctor–patient relationship firmly on the practitioner's side. A middle-aged housewife complaining of palpitations and intermittent bouts of a racing or thumping heart-beat might be alarmed to be told she had 'supraventricular tachycardia', or SVT. This merely means that her fast heart rate is coming from a signal in a part of the heart situated above the main muscular chambers. Simple. A teenage girl who faints while standing in the crowd at a pop concert, or an elderly man who faints when he gets up in the night to empty his bladder, might be terrified to hear that she or he had had a 'vasovagal episode' or an attack of 'micturition syncopy', respectively, but the words merely refer to the drop in blood pressure provoked by the consequences of their activity, resulting in a fall to the ground. Equally simple. A runner diagnosed with 'plantar fasciitis' might conceivably fear he will never don track shoes again, but he would soon be relieved to hear that he is only suffering from 'policeman's heel' or inflammation of the tendon in that area. Whilst acknowledging that in practice there are a few isolated instances where keeping the precise diagnosis from the patient is appropriate and in the best interests of that patient, by and large this conspiracy of linguistically induced terror is extremely damaging. If it had any place in clinical medicine it can surely be only as a dramatic device to heighten tension in fictitious TV dramas such as *Chicago Hope*, *ER* and *Casualty*, where medical abbreviations and euphemisms liberally pepper the script.

Nowhere is incomprehensible doctor-speak more potentially damaging than in circumstances where serious conditions like cancers are under discussion. Medics have somehow evolved a whole new language related to cancer, designed entirely to keep the patient in the dark for as long as possible. The euphemisms for the diagnostic label of cancer are numerous: malignancy, neoplasm, mitotic lesion, tumour, new growth, metastasis, carcinoma, rodent ulcer. Call it what you will, it is always cancer in some shape or form at the end of the day, and in most cases the patient would generally like to know. Paradoxically, these medical euphemisms which often act as obstacles to good doctor–patient communication are intriguing and exciting to many people. No sooner have they learned the jargon themselves, as patients, than they are proudly bandying the same terminology around the pub, the office or amongst their relatives in the expectation of attracting the same sense of awe and admiration as the doctors themselves attracted from them. It is bizarre. Patients interviewed by me on the TV sofa have often already become so conversant with their condition and its medical description that it is left to me to remind them of the need to explain in layman's terms, what they are saying rather than relying on their newly acquired medical expertise.

Poor Communication

When doctors do have to communicate in plain English, some find it depressingly difficult. This is especially so when it comes to breaking bad news and dealing with bereavement. Things are improving again without a doubt, but it is a sad reflection of the changes that have occurred in clinical practice over the past half century that special training is now necessary to teach doctors how to talk about difficult subjects when patients most need their support and therapeutic touch. Here, once again, their rigidly scientific approach tends to get in the way. It is too brutally honest to be gentle, too statistically accurate to be less than ruthless, and too unwaveringly objective to allow the recipient room for unjustified hope and optimism. A patient facing serious or terminal illness often has a need to believe in 'the special case', 'the miracle cure' and 'defiance of the odds'. But when hope is dashed, it may lead to despair, and if chronically and terminally ill patients are discouraged from believing in some mystical power or some vital supernatural force, if people who are bedridden or in constant pain are distracted from their faith, they can often just turn their faces to the wall and die. So while medical messages certainly need to be accurate and realistic, they also need to incorporate hope and comfort. Commonly used phrases, like 'there is nothing further we can do' and 'we simply don't know what causes this', leave too many questions unanswered and also give the impression that the doctor does not care and, in effect, is washing his hands of the whole problem. Patients often need to feel there is a reason for their predicament, just as someone who is recently bereaved constantly wonders, 'If only I had done something differently maybe his death would not have happened.' Few people really want to accept that they have become ill simply at random, by pure, cruel, unpredictable chance.

Medical communication can certainly remain accurate without being so brutally frank and inflexible. Even when death itself is a close and inevitable outcome, appropriate words can be a powerful and significant tool with which to prepare someone for what is to come. Complementary therapists are generally better equipped to offer their clients hope, promise and belief. They may not be in a position to guarantee a favourable outcome for the patient, or even hint at it, but patients certainly respond to an optimistic approach. So why is there such a difference in the way conventional and complementary therapists talk to patients about the likely outcome of their illnesses? One of the reasons may well be that conventional doctors are duty-bound to pass on any information they are asked for exactly as they understand it. Not to do so would be legally irresponsible. Complementary therapists, on the other hand, work with less information in the first place and cannot accurately gauge how their client will respond to their treatment, as little research evidence exists to support them. There is little risk of complementary therapists being subjected to litigation if they get it wrong.

The Depersonalization of the Patient

Another factor working against the establishment of warmer relationships between doctors and patients is the centralization and compartmentalization of health care in our large characterless modern hospitals. Patients who are already exposed and vulnerable because of their illness are rendered even more so as a result of their passive role in their impersonal hospital beds. Being ushered along endless hospital corridors towards more faceless departments, wearing no more than a flimsy gown, leaves most people feeling embarrassed and undignified. They are separated from their family and friends and have to rely on allocated visiting times to renew their links with their normal lives outside. Depersonalizing as this is for the patient, it also makes some aspects of the doctor's job more difficult, too. Information about how the patient lives, what his or her lifestyle consists of, and what the family dynamics are like, can be extremely useful in deciding how best to manage a person's medical or psychosocial problems. Dealing with patients in their home environment, as many GPs know, often strongly influences what treatment is selected, and who can best act as main carer.

Most complementary therapists have the advantage of seeing those of their clients who are less ill and not in need of hospital care in much warmer, cosier and less threatening environments which are more conducive to easy and relaxed consultations. Such consultations are much more likely to reveal intimate but crucial pointers to the real underlying cause of any partially diagnosed problem. However, even when complementary therapies are utilized within hospitals, as many indeed are in these enlightened times, the more personal, holistic approach is extremely useful in offsetting many of the cold, stark realities of the hospital ward, the urinary catheter or the bedpan.

Doctors as Patients

Doctors often only begin to recognize the isolating remoteness of modern medicine when they have the misfortune to become patients themselves. Suddenly they are made acutely aware of what it is like to be on the receiving end of treatment and, for most, it is a humbling and sobering experience. Medical journals are full of articles written by doctors flabbergasted by the impact that having the role of patient thrust upon them can have. They simply had no idea what it was like to be an ill person; they had never put themselves in the patient's shoes.

The culture shock of being suddenly transformed from the

decisive and commanding doctor to the unconfident passive patient was in fact immortalized in the excellent film *The Doctor*, starring William Hurt, in which a brilliant but brash and arrogant surgeon develops laryngeal cancer and embarks upon an incredibly steep learning curve of humility. The film concludes with him arranging to admit his healthy but equally arrogant medical students to hospital as patients for one whole weekend so that they may gain the most useful experience of their entire medical training – that of being a patient. Many of today's doctors would do well to see this film, and take on board its humbling message. Perhaps it should even become compulsory viewing for undergraduates.

The personal experience of illness is so powerful that doctors often return to the practice of medicine from their sickbeds with a totally altered attitude towards their patients. Many a paediatrician or obstetrician is a better and more rounded doctor for becoming a parent themselves, and any physician who has had their appendix out, slipped a disc or suffered the ignominy of uncontrolled diarrhoea, is that bit more likely to empathize with a similarly afflicted patient.

Whatever Happened to Empathy and Caring?

Since empathy is another quality which conventional medical training would do well to enhance, you would think that medical students and vocational trainees would be actively encouraged to express their feelings towards patients. Amazingly, this is not the case, and in fact doctors are deliberately trained *not* to show their feelings. Objectivity is all; to allow one's feelings and emotions into the equation, it is taught, is to get in the way of rational scientific thought. It is, in fact, for this very reason that doctors are discouraged from looking after and treating their own family's medical problems. However, while it is difficult to know exactly how to treat one's own wife, son or daughter because we love them so much, it should not be difficult to show some warmth and sympathy to patients we hardly know just because they are not family.

Vocationally trained GP clones, produced in recent years,

devoid, as they often appear, of normal feelings, may provoke dissatisfaction and distress in their patients for this reason, but doctors who seem to care and take trouble to express their emotions may do more for their patients in this way than with any of the sophisticated potions and pills they might offer. One of the greatest compliments a doctor can pay to a grieving family is to admit that they had become extremely fond of the person who has recently died. Some form of caring and personal obituary from the doctor can go a long way. The purely objective doctor, on the other hand, might precisely certify death, collect any unused medicines from the bedside table and hurry off to the next appointment. The true carer would spend time reminiscing with the bereaved family, talking over any remaining doubts or queries, giving them strength by congratulating them on the care and love they have provided, saying how well and courageously the deceased fought, and expressing sorrow and regret at their demise. A good GP, one that had known the family for a long time and come through thick and thin with them, might even divorce themselves from the super-efficient and totally objective medical clones and shed a tear or two. It really would not hurt, yet so many conventional doctors remain apparently aloof and distant from the feelings of others. In this regard they could learn a great deal from the naturally empathetic but less scientific body of complementary therapists.

Iatrogenic Illness

Iatrogenic illness is illness which has been caused by doctors or their treatments. For many this might seem a strange concept since doctors are the very people who are meant to cure disease, but the staggering truth is that some 10–30 per cent of hospital admissions may be due to iatrogenic illness. Two huge volumes entitled *Iatrogenic Diseases* (Oxford Medical Publications) are devoted entirely to illnesses brought about by conventional medical treatments. According to Lynne McTaggart, author of the book *What Doctors Don't Tell You*, each year 1.7 million people, a population the size of Birmingham, are put in a hospital bed simply by a procedure that has gone wrong.

Many will remember the damage caused by thalidomide. This was a drug marketed as an antiemetic (anti-sickness medication) but it was subsequently found to produce severe foetal abnormalities when taken by pregnant women. Opren was a drug aggressively publicized as a cure for arthritis, but it produced far more side effects in those that took it than the marketing had originally suggested. Tranquillizers, like diazepam (Valium) and its analogues, certainly had a place in medical treatment, and still do, but few would disagree that they were massively overprescribed following their launch, and that doctors are still now dealing with the awful results of iatrogenic addiction to these products. Slimming pills, once thought by many to be the quick-fix solution for anyone wanting to shed a few pounds in weight the easy way, have now been partially withdrawn because some of them have been found to be capable of damaging the valves of the heart even many years after the patient first took them. Even commonly used drugs that can be bought over the counter at the chemist, like aspirin and antihistamines, can cause problems, including bleeding from the stomach and daytime drowsiness respectively.

When more than one medicine is taken at a time, the risk of causing rather than solving problems becomes even greater. Many patients today take cocktails of prescribed medications, all of which are designed to achieve different results. The trouble is, such polypharmacy made the likelihood of a drug interaction that much more likely. Each drug is capable of potentiating or inhibiting the next. Desirable clinical effects are therefore over- or under-done. Patients taking warfarin, for example, to stop their blood clotting too quickly, might have a haemorrhage if the effect of the warfarin were enhanced, or a thrombosis if the effect were reduced. In either case, the consequence for the patient might be a stroke. Since each and every drug ever known to man carries risks, doctors with all these powerful pharmacological agents at their disposal have to be extremely careful to use them only where it is appropriate, and where any benefit vastly outweighs the risk. In the past, this has not always been the case.

Conventional doctors may produce iatrogenic illness in other ways. Excessive doses of radiotherapy and routine vaccination can bring about rare but catastrophic results. The subsequent publicity leaves a deep, enduring apprehension in the minds of the public concerning these procedures, and all too often the benefits of such preventative therapy, as indeed it is intended to be, are completely forgotten. National organizations, like RAGE (Radiotherapy Action Group Exposure) and JABS (Justice, Awareness and Basic Support) have been specifically set up to raise public awareness of these issues. Both have important questions to pose doctors but both must be careful not to poison the minds of potential patients against the appropriate use of such therapies.

Surgery, too, can occasionally produce unpredictable problems. It is easy to forget how many lives are extended or saved through modern surgery, and all too easy to remember a case or instance when an operation seemed to be the beginning of someone's problem rather than the end of it. Keloid scars, wound and chest infections, deep vein thromboses, even death under anaesthetic – all are rare but occasional consequences of surgery that may or may not have been avoidable, but will always remain theoretical possibilities with treatments as invasive and critical as this. Complementary therapists, with their massage oils, acupuncture needles and herbal supplements, are not faced with comparably hazardous dangers.

Medical Negligence and Defensive Medicine

The development of an iatrogenic condition does not necessarily signify any lack of care or knowledge on the part of the doctor. In fact, many treatments, for example antidepressants, are almost certain to produce minor side effects in order to achieve the clinical benefits they are designed to bestow. These are iatrogenic effects, but necessary ones and ones for which the doctor should in no way be blamed. But true medical negligence seems to be becoming much more common, with more than one-third of senior doctors now being sued at some stage of their careers.

According to the British Medical Association, being sued by aggrieved patients is now becoming something of an occupational hazard for hospital doctors, and the Royal College of General Practitioners is equally concerned that the same is true of general practice. The Medical Defence Union states that the number of medical negligence cases brought, and the amount of money awarded, has risen at an average rate of 15 per cent a year in the last five years. Consequently, the amount the NHS pays out in compensation is steadily rising, and in 1998 is expected to top £250 million per annum. Although the majority of doctors are subsequently exonerated from such claims of negligence, this is a worrying trend. There are many reasons for it, although I would not include among them that doctors are practising an inferior brand of medical care.

A study conducted by the Medical Protection Society in the 1980s found that only one in eight patients who would have had a case for compensation actually ever bothered to sue. The difference is that now people are no longer content to put complete trust in a professional, and are much more likely to question a doctor's competence. With huge sums of money being awarded in successful cases, the financial incentive to bring cases before the courts has also increased. There are also many people who genuinely want to make sure that what has happened to them never happens to anyone else.

As I have explained earlier, an unfortunate consequence of the rising numbers of medical negligence cases is an increase in the practice of defensive medicine. This means that, in some cases, patients might be over-investigated for fear that something incredibly unlikely might be missed, and, in other cases, that high risk procedures will be avoided because of the risk of any potentially harmful side effects. Taken to an extreme, such defensive practices would result in no patient ever finding a doctor willing to conduct a coronary bypass graft, no mother-to-be finding a doctor happy to supervise childbirth at home, and no physician ever performing a lumbar puncture for suspected meningitis.

Trial by Media

The media, who have done so much to publicize every medical scandal of recent times, should be careful to balance their stories to reflect what usually happens in Britain's general practice surgeries. If we only read about the wrong operation being done on the wrong patient, that doctors are still playing God, that another drug has been withdrawn because of its side effects, that the medical profession itself has been pushing dangerous slimming pills, that cervical smear recalls have had to be set up because women are dying from cancer who were given the all-clear, that many a diagnosis of meningitis has been missed, and that another patient has been sent all around the country when no available bed was ready for him, no sensible patient would ever take his symptoms to a conventionally trained doctor. Most people, however, have a higher regard for the orthodox medical profession than this, and current surveys reveal that over 80 per cent of patients are entirely satisfied with the efforts of their NHS doctors.

Openness and Honesty

Several NHS trusts are now employing 'risk managers' to deal with potential claimants and to avoid future mistakes, and better record-keeping, improved supervision of junior staff and reduced workloads are needed. But improved communications are the key to reducing medical negligence cases. If doctors are granted enough time and take enough trouble to explain to patients exactly what is proposed for their treatment, and what the possible benefits and risks are, and are also able to bring the patient into the decision making process fewer of these claims would ever come the doctor's way. Furthermore, even when mistakes are made, if doctors could only find it in themselves to say the simple word 'sorry', then the vast majority of complaints would simply melt away.

Patients are aware that medicine can be a high-risk profession and that doctors are often overworked and stressed. They also understand that doctors are human beings and capable of error. They tend to become angry and litigious only when they sniff any hint of a cover-up, or when a guilty doctor fails to apologize for his mistake. Doctors are much less likely to close ranks and defend each other than they used to be and many specialists know that they can double their incomes through the legal profession by specifically contradicting any stance taken by their rival specialist in the dock. This modern scenario, in which doctors are happy and willing to speak out against each other, will no doubt increasingly blur the boundaries of what is generally considered good or negligent practice. Some law firms even advertise for patients on a nationwide basis, trawling for people who feel that they may have been harmed by their doctors. The longer these trends in the legal profession are allowed to continue, the more dissatisfied the general population is likely to become with the medical profession.

Medical Uncertainties Brought About by 'Progress'

Not very long ago, medical treatment revolved around a small number of accepted certainties: penicillin would cure a straightforward pneumonia; insulin would treat a diabetic; surgery would be the obvious treatment for somebody suffering from a stomach ulcer. Now, an alternative and more recently developed antibiotic might be more appropriate than penicillin, different formulations of insulin can be tailored to the individual diabetic's needs, and the mainline therapy for stomach ulcers is a course of 'triple therapy' involving the use of three separate drugs to eradicate the organism *Helicobacter Pylori* from the lining of the stomach.

Things have changed, and in the process have become so much more complex that modern medical treatment is as confusing as it is sophisticated. Where once we were told that all cholesterol was bad and harmful, now we are told that there are such things as good cholesterol and bad cholesterol. Where once we were told by educational psychologists that difficult children required increased discipline, now we are told that the underlying cause may be attention deficit hyperactivity disorder or dyslexia, which require far more subtle and appropriate handling. Having been told that the new antidepressant agents were the best thing since sliced bread, now we are warned that they may lead to suicide attempts and severe behavioural changes within the first fortnight of use. There is uncertainty about the clinical benefits of screening men for prostate cancer, and the argument rages over whether breast screening for all women is really cost-effective or whether prophylactic hormonal treatment in 'at-risk' women would save more lives for less money. Controversy and debate have polarized people, who have developed their own opinions and prejudices. When different doctors say so many contradictory things, it is hardly surprising that attitudes to orthodox medical practices have become less trusting and a great deal more circumspect.

Patient Power

In the last few years there has been increased emphasis on 'patient power'. This has been partly set up by government initiatives to increase personal responsibility amongst members of the public towards their own health, and includes directives in the Patient's Charter, which establishes a number of rights and privileges for patients. Medical education and increasingly accessible health services have empowered larger numbers of people to demand superior health care, and to become much more active than they used to be in obtaining the appropriate treatment. That these measures have become necessary at all bears witness to the fact that for too long doctors contrived to retain the balance of power in medical transactions, and attempted to keep the patient relatively ill-informed as to the true situation. Too many patients underwent operations without fully understanding why they were necessary or what the likely outcome would be; too few ever gave informed consent. All of this has now changed thanks to 'patient power'.

Patients also recognize that doctors are only human and that, as such, they have different approaches and attitudes. They realize that they should be able to select the doctor of their choice, and to say that they are not satisfied with the opinions of one over another. They are less likely now to accept gloomy prognoses from one specialist without at least seeking another opinion from a different specialist. Where some surgeons will never contemplate a given procedure, others will enthusiastically take it on, and where some offer no hope to the terminally or chronically ill, others will gladly do what they can to make the remainder of their patients' lives more fulfilling. The phrase, 'Trust me, I'm a doctor' has therefore been considerably watered down in the light of this increasing medical knowledge, and it has left the lay public with the distinct impression that patients must shop around for good, trustworthy medical care.

Medical Politics

While it is true that politicians have created benefits for patients, they have also created worries. In Britain, the NHS has been converted into a kind of political football and is constantly under threat of disintegration and possible dismantling. The developments in fundholding general practice introduced in the last 10 years or so (where family doctors were made responsible for their own budgets), in practice formularies (where doctors were only allowed to prescribe from a limited medicines list), and in item-for-service payments (like monetary rewards or vaccination quotas), have left the public wondering whether the services they were once guaranteed are being squeezed and restricted beyond their control.

Hospital managers still have to decide whether certain forms of treatment will be made available or not. Will a patient with relapsing multiple sclerosis, for example, be able to receive the expensive new drug beta-interferon in the particular region in which he or she lives? (Theoretically, this drug could reduce the patient's frequency of symptom relapses by up to a third.) Will an otherwise fit gentleman of 62 be able to have a coronary artery bypass graft or a kidney transplant? And will hundreds of infertile couples be eligible for infertility treatment in any given area? Doctors have had to compete with one another in order to place a sick patient in a hospital bed, and rely on special care baby units sometimes exclusively supported by charitable donations in order to keep premature babies alive. Patients are sometimes refused operations simply because of their age. Is it really surprising that anger and resentment are heaped upon the medical profession for allowing this to happen?

Government funding has also been criticized because of its prejudicial emphasis regarding expenditure. Breast cancer accounts for 15,000 deaths a year and attracts £8 million in research funds against a mere £400,000 for cancer of the prostate which is responsible for 9,500 deaths per year. And although most women are screened for breast and cervical cancer, awareness of and screening for male cancers are rare. Women, in fact, use nearly two-thirds of all GP and NHS resources.

Who Controls the Doctors?

There has always been a code of conduct and behaviour on which relationships between doctors and patients, and between different doctors, are founded. Ethical standards in Britain are generally enforced by the General Medical Council, who keep a watching brief on a wide range of professional behaviour, including the involvement of doctors with patients and their families, their clinical competence, public image and commercial activity. Areas in which medical ethics are particularly important are confidentiality and obtaining informed consent from patients.

The conduct of doctors who enrol patients in research studies is as strictly controlled as it is in the care of the dying, in termination of pregnancy, in the care of patients with mental disorders, and in preventing sick doctors from practising. Interestingly, medical ethics also prevent conventional doctors from referring their patients to unlicensed practitioners of complementary medicine. But the public understanding of which medical ethics are acceptable and which are not has been stretched and challenged in recent years. Many feel that the doctors' governing body's interpretation of the rules pertaining to euthanasia is inadequate, and that the area is poorly policed. Some are critical of developments in the world of fertility treatments, where some deserving individuals are left without help while others are assisted in having a child through artificial means at the age of 60, and where frozen embryos may be used in medical experimentation or sold to any third party wealthy enough to pay for them. In the USA, feelings have run so high over the abortion issue that gynaecologists have been gunned down outside their clinics, and in Britain, similarly strong feelings are expressed whenever a patient diagnosed as being in a permanent vegetative state has his or her life support machine switched off.

Many considerations are also involved in the increasingly significant but complex area of genetic research. On the one hand, this promises to find not just a treatment but a cure for the hundreds of congenital and hereditary diseases which affect both the quantity and quality of thousands of sufferers' lives. On the other hand, it has the potential to alter the genetic make-up of the individual permanently, and to tamper with the very fabric of heredity itself It was only just over 50 years ago that German doctors and scientists were involved with the Nazis' 'final solution' and other forms of unethical and deadly human experimentation; no doubt if they had had access to human genetic engineering at the time, they would certainly have used it for their own appalling purposes. It is understandable, therefore, that worries that unregulated genetic scientists might experiment on defenceless frozen embryos, as they are already doing on living animals in some institutions, leave some people angry and horrified. Most can see that ethical experimentation has much to offer the human race, just as genetic engineering enabled insulin to be synthetically made so the lives of those suffering from diabetes could be saved. But all work must be rigidly and ethically controlled, and be backed at the end of the day by popular public opinion.

Modern Medicine in Crisis

Despite all the marvellous achievements that have taken place throughout the last century, an atmosphere of apprehension and doubt now pervades medicine. The euphoric bubble created with penicillin, with organ transplantation and with the birth of Louise Brown, the world's first 'test-tube baby', has burst, and medicine has now become much more vulnerable to criticism. The above limitations of conventional care, the financial rationing of scientific medicine and the slowing down of research in important and emotive areas, such as cancer, Alzheimer's disease, schizophrenia and other degenerative diseases, have created huge doubts for the future. Unrealistically high expectations have not been realized, and many people are questioning the direction in which modern medicine is actually going. When will the striving to keep people alive for as long as possible, whatever their circumstances, ever stop? How far will patients be excluded from treatment simply because of age, money or whether they smoke or not? And has medicine just become a service industry, existing purely to satisfy whatever fantasies its patients want fulfilled – a breast enhancement, a nose job or a face-lift, for example? The orthodox medical profession has even resorted to perfecting therapies for normal life events such as the menopause and obesity, and to correcting non-specific and relatively trivial complaints, like snoring, with intricate and sometimes esoteric procedures. The attitude of 'can do, must do' has got out of hand and it has become popular to believe that every single person suffers from some condition or another, and that everyone can be relieved of it through treatment. In view of all this, it is imperative that conventional medicine recognizes its limitations and decides, with broad agreement of both professional and lay opinion, in which direction it is heading. Many of the doubts and uncertainties may be resolved through the efforts of a commonsense ethics committee and through trust and common decency. This it must do if it is to return once more to the basic philosophical aims of Hippocrates. In doing so, it will need to borrow many of the good qualities found in complementary therapies.

CHAPTER 4

The Benefits of Alternative Medicine

Interest in alternative medicine and the popularity of complementary therapies are booming. In the last 10 years, vastly increasing numbers of people have turned to sources of healing beyond the realms of recognized conventional treatment. One-seventh of the British population did so a decade ago, and now this number has swelled to one-quarter. Some 4 million visits are now paid every year to practitioners of complementary therapy, and the number of therapists is growing by over 10 per cent annually. In other parts of the world, especially America, France and Australia, people are even more enthusiastic about alternative medicine than they are in Britain.

Clearly, complementary medicine has something to offer that orthodox practitioners of medicine are failing to deliver. Even GPs themselves are aware of this; in fact, in 1997, three-quarters of fundholding GPs stated that they would welcome the establishment of some kind of complementary practice within their own surgery premises. As long as GPs can remain politically able to control their own budgets, this is increasingly likely to happen, and in fact 30 per cent of GPs are currently offering complementary medical services to their patients, and many are actually delivering these services themselves. Many family doctors have learned the arts of hypnosis, acupuncture, homeopathy and other techniques, and several of their fraternity even regard themselves as spiritual healers. Other doctors have not gone so far as to incorporate these skills into their own therapeutic repertoire, but are happy to employ outside therapists to help in their busy clinics. The regulatory bodies which control the medical profession have also recently adopted a much less stand-offish approach to certain sections of complementary medicine. The very people who not so long ago made it illegal for a doctor to refer patients to any complementary therapist have now accepted that, provided the physician in charge of the patient maintains overall responsibility, complementary therapy can be practised under the NHS hand in hand with orthodox medicine.

Britain's first ever Chair in complementary medicine has now been set up at Exeter University under the auspices of Professor Edzard Ernst, whose task it is to evaluate its scientific validity and safety. Professor Ernst has already stated clearly that he is most interested in finding out whether complementary medicine is safe and whether or not it works. He is not so much concerned to discover whether orthodox doctors feel threatened, as some obviously do, but whether the public is adequately protected. Several protocols for approval by the University's Medical Research Ethics Committee are already being put together, but the final results of the studies are obviously some considerable time off. In the meantime, increasing numbers of people are toying with the idea of complementary therapy and increasing numbers of practitioners are willing to provide it for them. Certainly it has a lot to offer.

Dissatisfaction with Conventional Therapy

One of the reasons for the increasing popularity of complementary therapy is undoubtedly that large sections of the population have become dissatisfied and disillusioned with conventional medicine. People have been made increasingly aware of its drawbacks and limitations, and there is no longer the blind faith in it which existed up to 20 years ago following the honeymoon period in the 1950s and 1960s when it seemed as though conventional medicine could cure just about everything. The discovery that many common conditions *cannot* be cured by conventional treatment (in fact can be made worse by it), that different people with the same condition require different treatments, and that some healers have more to offer than others, has fuelled an intense interest in alternative medical practices which are often considered gentler, safer and more natural.

Gentle Medicine

One of the many attractions of complementary medicine is that it is a gentler form of therapy than most conventional treatments. Whilst potent and powerful modern drugs have undoubtedly saved lives in serious and life-threatening conditions, they also have the capacity to produce unpleasant and far-reaching side effects and adverse reactions when used inappropriately or for more trivial complaints. Complementary therapy, on the other hand, is perceived as kinder and gentler, with a much reduced risk of causing harm to those who use it. It is wholly right that would-be patients have learned to question the validity of pharmaceutical medicines prescribed by doctors who, all too often, are not entirely aware of all the possible consequences of and interaction pertaining to any given drug. For the subtler, vague and nebulous symptoms, which often form the bread-and-butter workload of the complementary therapist, a 'gentler' medicine is generally much preferred by the patient on the receiving end.

Natural Medicine

Unlike the synthetic, highly sophisticated and refined products utilized by doctors, the remedies and treatments used by complementary therapists are often derived from natural sources. Those subscribing to philosophies of medicine which embrace the concept of the continuity of man with Nature find this link compelling, and would always far rather exploit what Mother Nature has to offer by way of a healing cure first. Herbalists can boast that all their wares are God-given and remain untainted by the destructive hand of man. Aromatherapists merely tap into the wonderful fragrances and essences which living things create. Practitioners of manipulative techniques, such as chiropractic and reflexology, simply strive to restore the patient's body to full and normal function by physically adjusting joint alignment and posture, and calling upon those innate self-healing powers buried deep within. The attraction of avoiding the invasive methods of treatment employed by conventional doctors, and replacing them instead with the age-old goodness of what this planet has always provided, is an overwhelming and over-riding factor for many of the devotees of alternative medicine.

Safer Medicine

Since it has been estimated that a million British people are hospitalized each year by a conventional medical procedure that has gone wrong, and that no medicinal drug exists which is entirely free of all possible side effects, it is hardly surprising that complementary practices can also produce their own problems and occasionally cause harm to the patient. However, by and large, they involve treatments that are externally applied to the patient, in cases where the treatment is taken internally, the remedies used tend to be dilute, natural and essentially non-toxic.

A More Relaxed Approach

One of complementary medicine's major advantages is that the patient is able to spend much more time with the therapist than he is with the conventionally trained doctor. The average six minutes per patient that orthodox doctors are confined to is woefully inadequate, and I personally defy anybody to convince me that proper medicine can be practised with these kinds of time constraints. By contrast, complementary therapists are often able to devote up to one and a half hours to the first consultation with a client. The environment in which patients are seen is generally more cosy and relaxed, there is no waiting-room full of sick people outside, and the clients are given the time and opportunity to explain all their symptoms and complaints in depth, knowing that the therapist is likely to listen attentively and patiently to all they have to say without interruption. Following this, the therapist can enquire and probe further into lifestyle, relationship and occupational factors, and still have plenty of opportunity thereafter to explore the client's interpretation of their symptoms and to come to some mutual agreement about the proposed treatment. Orthodox doctors tend to place the patient in a passive role, deciding themselves which treatment is best, and rarely giving the patient any choice in the treatment plan. In complementary therapy, the client feels much more included in the consultation and is therefore much more likely to comply with the therapy offered.

The benefits of extended consultation time must not be underestimated. More often than not, patients with psychosocial problems above all else need someone to listen to them. The age-old adage that a problem shared is a problem halved still holds true, and in this busy world where people have all too little time to off-load their stresses and strains on to those better trained to deal with them, an hour and a half spent talking to someone who genuinely wants to hear is a great luxury. Clients often say they feel better already just for having spent that length of time voicing their problems. Sometimes they are problems that have never been discussed before. Indisputably, time is of the essence, and this is an area where complementary therapy has a definite advantage.

Paying for Treatment

In alternative medicine, the relationship between the healer and the client starts on a different footing, because generally the client is paying directly for the services he receives. Unlike the indirect route of payment throughout the NHS, where the government taxes everyone in employment and redistributes the money as it sees fit, most people seeing a healer are entering into a one-to-one financial transaction in which the client has made a definite choice and knows exactly what he is spending his money on.

It is possible that the direct handing over of money might be partly instrumental in any given patient's recovery. Depending on the individual, the mere act of spending cash can necessitate receiving value for money. Since the money is usually non-refundable, patients already have a vested interest in making sure they are going to feel better. Who knows how psychologically important it is to justify the expense of complementary therapy by convincing oneself that it is working? Who knows how easy it might be to dismiss conventional treatment as worthless, if it is perceived to be available free of charge whenever you want it?

The Patient in Control

In a complementary therapy situation, the relationship between the patient and the healer is generally such that the patient is in control of the treatment. The healer listens to what the patient feels about the cause of their symptoms and problems, and is less likely than the orthodox doctor to attempt to contradict the patient's interpretation. This often makes patients feel that the complementary therapist is more on their side. Lifestyle factors are much more likely to be taken into account, and a much greater proportion of the advice and treatment given by the therapist is devoted to suggested alternatives to the way patients lead their lives on an everyday basis.

Complementary practitioners also often appear to be more passionate and enthusiastic about their therapy. They are less cynical on the whole than conventional doctors, often believing absolutely in the ability of their chosen speciality to make clients better. Most complementary therapists adopt the type of lifestyle that they would recommend to their patients, and stick to it. They are also very good at addressing the fears and anxieties exhibited by their clients in order that a more positive mindset can be established. In similar ways, chronically ill patients and even the dying can obtain hope and optimism from alternative practitioners. The last thing such patients want to hear is 'I'm afraid there is nothing more I can do for you other than relieve your pain,' which is often the case in a conventional medical setting. Complementary therapists may not and should not give such patients cause to believe in a cure, but they are very able to make their patients' situations easier and more acceptable. They often appear more able to relieve the suffering and discomfort of such people by producing effects above and beyond those of strong analgesics and tranquillizers.

Empathy

Doctors themselves make very bad patients, usually because they tend either to fuss too much or too little over their condition. Some are stoics who stubbornly refuse to see another medical colleague even when they know they have potentially serious symptoms, feeling that they have somehow let themselves or their colleagues down. Others, at the opposite end of the scale, become quite hypochondriacal about the least little thing, regarding every headache as a potential brain tumour, every back pain as a slipped disc and every cough as evolving tuberculosis. But whenever doctors do become ill, their empathy levels towards their patients dramatically increase, at least in the short term. If only all doctors, like most complementary therapists, were able to put themselves in their patients' shoes. If only they could imagine what it must be like to be in their position. If only they could fully comprehend the implications, consequences and repercussions of every illness for every patient. How much more caring and sympathetic physicians and surgeons would be. Complementary therapists, on the other hand, are much better at empathizing with their clients. They tend to express their own emotions freely, unrestricted as they are from the imprisoning objectivity of a doctor's scientific training.

Consequently, patients are much more likely to hear phrases like 'I'm so sorry, that must be awful for you' and 'How are you coping?' from complementary therapists than from orthodox doctors.

Complementary therapists are also likely to be less judgemental in their approach than doctors, who are sometimes guilty of condemning patients for their actions, particularly if these have led to emotional, social or physical difficulties. Therapists are more inclined to work towards solutions to the problems. For example, a teenage girl seeking a termination of pregnancy is not helped by her GP foisting his or her own religious beliefs upon her; a young man with severe scarring acne is devastated at being told that his fatty diet has caused his problems; and the workaholic executive who has just had his first coronary is in no fit state to be informed that he brought his heart attack upon himself. By contrast, the philosophy of the alternative practitioner is to bolster patients emotionally until they are ready to accept that they have not been looking after themselves as well as they should. The next step is to motivate the patient to work in tandem with the therapist towards correcting unhealthy lifestyles.

Prevention Rather Than Cure

Until recently, conventional medicine was almost entirely disease orientated: patients were only expected to visit the doctor's surgery when they felt ill and developed symptoms. Anyone who went to the doctor when they weren't ill felt they were wasting the doctor's time. In the last 10 years, however, the medical profession has become more involved with health promotion and screening as a means of preventing illness, but by and large the achievement of 'well-being' and 'good health' has always been much more an objective of complementary therapists.

The philosophy of the alternative practitioner has always stated that health is much more than freedom from disease, and that a person's emotional, spiritual and physical being must remain in balance and harmony at all times. They believe that illness may be prevented by maintaining that equilibrium and that only when it is disturbed do symptoms emerge and illness become established. Orthodox doctors, on the other hand, are much happier to believe in the randomness of disease, and are relatively uninterested in whether their patients' problems have an emotional, physical or spiritual basis. This is one of the fundamental differences between the two philosophies, and partly explains why, in a country where major infectious epidemics are no longer a threat and public health is good that complementary therapy is gaining in popularity. The more subtle and nebulous complaints brought about by a physically healthier but spiritually poorer world population, are better suited to the skills of complementary practitioners than orthodox doctors who remain disease-orientated clinicians.

Orthodox doctors may search at length for a physical diagnosis of illness in a patient with inexplicable symptoms, but are powerless to act when one cannot be found. Their complementary counterparts, on the other hand, are entirely happy to work without any definitive diagnosis on the basis that the patient's condition may entirely be generated by the patient's environment and lifestyle. There is now the growing belief that it is not enough just to be 'healthy' – one should also feel well. Consequently, in order to enhance well-being and self-esteem, and to maximize one's true potential, many people now seek the services of an appropriate complementary therapist.

The Appeal of the Traditional

Another major attraction of complementary therapy is its simple, ancient and traditional philosophy. In our modern world with its huge appetite for fresh ideas and concepts, the exotic and trans-cultural pull of weird and wonderful esoteric remedies is irresistible. Many of the conventional medical philosophies remain incomprehensible and complex to the average person, but there is a fundamental and unifying purity and homogeneity in the philosophies on which most complementary therapies are based. Amongst them is the idea of a continuity between man and nature. Just as our ancestors believed so many people today still believe we are closely related to all other animal species, and that we can adopt many of their individual characteristics, for example the wisdom of the owl, the strength and courage of a lion or the freedom of a bird. For many, the affinity between mankind and the animal kingdom, which is exploited in many alternative philosophies, is essential.

Vitalistic or life-force theories are central to most complementary practices, and are based on the fact that the spirit or life-force is the single factor distinguishing a living being from its identical-looking dead shell. The life-force can take various forms according to your beliefs – an independent fluid or miasma, an aura around the body, or energy pathways running vertically down the body – but the ability to influence the life-force remains a concept with which most people can readily identify. The doctrine of similarities has also proved simple and effective. Since a bull is noted for its strength and power, its blood might be utilized to confer potency and strength to anyone who drank it. A yellow bird might be sacrificed in an attempt to cure somebody of jaundice.

The contagion theory runs central to the practice of witchcraft and is based on the concept of magical connections between objects that share certain attributes. In voodoo, this suggests that any part of a person can be manipulated, even from some considerable distance, to influence the rest of the person. In much the same way, and to achieve much the same effect, soldiers in some societies would thrust a weapon that had been used in battle into a fire in the hope and expectation of further adding to the agonies and wounds of those who had been cut by it.

These very early concepts, which were often fervently upheld by primitive man, were superseded by the philosophies of Hippocrates and the ancient Chinese, who introduced a more structured, rational and holistic approach to medicine. Hippocrates believed that health was the result of a balance between the various 'humours', consisting of earth, water, fire and air, and that any disequilibrium in these humours would result in disease. He, like the ancient Chinese, treated patients as individuals, paying attention not only to their physical health, but also to their emotional and spiritual well-being. Thus, although he was the first scientific empiricist, setting up sophisticated and meticulous medical documentation for his prescribed treatments, he was also a fervent believer in the holistic approach.

The Belief in Self-Healing

Many complementary therapists believe in the power of self-healing, the ability of the individual to heal from within. This is an extension of the life-force belief and derives its evidence from the fact that the body recovers without help from colds, wounds and cuts, and broken limbs. According to this philosophy, when the healing process becomes blocked or inhibited, disease will manifest itself, sometimes even in the form of serious illness or cancer. By stimulating the healing process, therapists claim that cancer antibodies, for example, might be created, thereby neutralizing and eradicating the origin of the illness.

Whether self-healing as a concept is real or merely a metaphor for the human spirit is irrelevant to thousands of people who believe that health comes from within. Conventional doctors may often question these beliefs, but complementary therapists will generally accept them.

Treating the Individual

Complementary therapists are much more likely than orthodox doctors to treat different patients with the same condition differently. The treatment, they say, must be tailored to individual needs as each person will produce symptoms and signs unique to them, and react differently to any given set of circumstances. Homeopaths stress that the prescriptions they make up are always selected with the individual in mind, and practitioners of traditional Chinese herbalism follow similar principles. Conventional doctors, on the other hand, generally attempt to categorize patients under the names of diseases and tend to treat the disease rather than the individual. For a while, patients themselves began to believe that there was one pill for every ill, but things have changed in the last 20 years, and patients are now inclined to seek different potencies, types and frequencies of treatment according to their character and circumstances. Such patients are more likely to derive satisfaction from complementary rather than conventional therapies.

Taking Personal Responsibility

Fewer people today are prepared to put their trust entirely in the hands of their doctors. The government itself has been encouraging the population to take more responsibility for its own health, and few would disagree that those of us who are best informed and medically educated will press for and receive the best medical care. Complementary therapy is well placed to give patients that personal responsibility because clients take a much more active role in making decisions about their treatment. Moreover, they do not wait until they are ill before visiting the doctor, or until they receive a screening recall letter; they go before they develop symptoms or when they want to boost their well-being and overall level of health. This would be difficult or impossible to achieve in the surgeries of most family doctors.

The Holistic Approach

Although a handful of Britain's doctors can congratulate themselves on practising true holistic medicine, this approach is much more common within the realms of complementary medicine. It is one of the most important reasons why so many thousands of people are now flocking to practitioners of alternative medicine, and away from the reductionist attitudes of conventional doctors. Therapists who take a holistic approach regard each patient as a whole entity, and see individuals as unique. This avoids the conventional process of categorizing patients according to their disease, and allows for different perspectives and more than one single truth. It enables the therapist to respond to people in terms of their body, mind and spirit within the context of their family, their culture and their environment. In addition, a holistic approach can be applied to a wide variety of therapies, including drugs and surgery, but also embracing meditation, diet, massage and manipulation. In holistic therapy, concrete emphasis is placed on the patient's role in the relationship between the patient and the therapist, and there is also an implied awareness of the importance of the health of the practitioner as well as the patient. The 'Physician heal thyself' is central to the whole concept of holism, and the original Hippocratic oath is founded largely on the mind–spirit–body link. Regrettably, many conventional doctors have only paid lip service to it in the last half century, allowing complementary therapists to espouse its principles almost exclusively.

Alternative as Anti-Establishment

Promoters of alternative health care often gain public sympathy by portraying themselves as a beleaguered minority fighting a self-serving monolithic establishment. For those who have increasingly tended to reject science as a method of determining truth, and whose distrust of doctors and medical technology has grown, the underdog role which complementary therapy has adopted is yet another of its attractions. The implied threat to the conventional profession can be gauged by the measure of their loathing for it and only convinces the alternative brethren further of the deep-seated inadequacy of the orthodox approach.

Miracle Cures

Anecdotal evidence that complementary therapy has rescued patients from the jaws of death abounds, and has undoubtedly fuelled the growing interest and curiosity in its capabilities. Because complementary therapy is relatively new in Britain, it has received a very favourable press from journalists who have been happy to hype such human-interest stories and boost their newspaper's circulation figures. But human-interest stories speak for themselves. If hundreds upon hundreds of individuals have come forward, all testifying to the efficacy and power of alternative medical practices, the rest of the population can only ignore them up to a point. Sooner or later the impression becomes ingrained that here is a true and viable alternative to conventional medicine which can offer considerable advantages, and can even result in medical recoveries which defy scientific explanation. The testimonials of all of those recipients of complementary medicine who have contributed their personal view of the therapies covered in Chapter 6 of this book are just the tip of the iceberg. Hundreds and thousands of people are convinced that complementary therapy works, and thousands more turn to its practitioners every year. Whether patients merely *believe* they feel better, or actually do get better is almost irrelevant. The fact that there is a subjective improvement in well-being and symptomatology speaks volumes and will ensure the increasing and accelerating popularity of alternative medicine.

Scientific Proof

Although, in many instances, it is difficult to carry out scientific trials on complementary therapies, they can and have been undertaken. However, some practitioners actively reject any attempt at statistical evaluation on the basis that the treatment in which they are involved is beyond science; others claim they simply do not have the financial means or know-how to embark on such studies; and, for many, the fact that such a large proportion of their patients subjectively feel better and are happy to continue with their treatment and to pay for such treatment, is sufficient. But complementary therapy will never be accepted by the conventional medical fraternity, and never fully incorporated into and paid for by the NHS, until it is capable of showing that it has a proven place in the therapeutic armoury against ill-health.

The good news is that, over the years, evidence has accumulated which demonstrates that many of the main complementary therapies can be proved to be effective for at least certain conditions. For example: chiropractic techniques have been shown to be more effective in the treatment of low back pain than conventional medical care carried out in orthopaedic out-patient departments; studies have shown that acupuncture can affect animals as well as humans, even those under anaesthetic, lending further weight to the claim that acupuncture works on a physical level, not just because people believe in it; reports in the *British Medical Journal* have shown that 81 out of 105 scientific trials on homeopathy were positive; psychiatrists have now accepted that St John's wort (Hypericum) is an effective herbal treatment for depression; hypnotherapists have impressively demonstrated their skills in treating asthma, irritable bowel syndrome and certain types of recurrent headache; elimination diets have helped people with rheumatoid arthritis and migraine, and vastly improved in some cases the behavioural difficulties experienced in hyperactive children. Other trials, too numerous to mention here but documented in Chapter 6 of this book have lent weight to the tolerability and efficacy of many complementary therapies. However, there are many others with no scientific evidence whatsoever with which to substantiate their claims, and while their clients continue to seem, for the large part, unconcerned about the need for such substantiation, it is unlikely the situation will change. Nevertheless, there is a moral and ethical requirement to demonstrate in some meaningful way that any so-called therapy is worthwhile, not only in terms of money and time, but in emotional and spiritual ways as well. The Council for Complementary and Alternative Medicine recognizes these requirements, and realizes that complementary medicine can only expand and flourish if it pushes ahead with the regulation and evaluation of its own practices. Greater efforts to prove its value will inevitably follow.

Royal Approval

Prince Charles and the entire royal family carry homeopathic medicines with them wherever they go, and their physicians have also chosen to train in various alternative techniques, including osteopathy and acupuncture. The Prince is quoted as saying 'I am personally convinced that many people could benefit from complementary medicine. It is also clear from the enormous increase in complementary therapies used by the general public, largely paid for out of their own pockets, that I am not entirely alone in that belief. It would appear that we have reached a defining moment in our attitude towards health care in this country among the public and health care professionals.' When the future King of England speaks out and encourages the modern NHS to embrace medicine and techniques from all cultures, people sit up and take notice. They certainly did when, in October 1997, he spoke at St James's Palace in celebration of the centenary of the King's Fund, of which he is President: 'There is,' he said, 'a feeling, not only among patients but also among GPs, nurses and other mainstream health practitioners, that there needs to be greater integration and interprofessional collaboration in patient care, and that we can each as individuals play a greater role in contributing towards our own health and well-being.' At the same time, Prince Charles was aware that what he was saying was controversial, and that certain sections of the medical profession remained frankly antagonistic. 'The goal we must work towards,' he went on, 'is an integrated health care system in which all the knowledge, wisdom and experience accumulated in different ways, at different times and in different cultures is effectively deployed to prevent or alleviate human suffering.' The Prince's sentiments at the time were mirrored by many others encouraged by the cautious welcome the British Medical Association had granted the growth of alternative medicine. Indeed, the BMA's own report, *Complementary Medicine: New Approaches to Good Practice*, published in 1993, and a General Medical Council report entitled *Tomorrow's Doctor*, published the same year, reflected the increasing changes in attitude. With the gradual thawing of resistance amongst even the most die-hard and entrenched medical views, it seems that complementary therapy will become ever more popular.

CHAPTER 5

The Limitations of Alternative Medicine

Regulatory Problems

Complementary medicine is an extremely broad area encompassing as it does the Eastern therapies, including acupuncture, Chinese herbalism and ayurvedic medicine, with manipulative therapies such as chiropractic, osteopathy and reflexology. It includes aromatherapy, homeopathy and other natural therapies, and active therapies such as the Alexander technique, hypnotherapy and yoga. It even includes the miscellaneous therapies involving external powers, like spiritual healing, crystal therapy and radionics. Some are genuine alternatives to conventional medicine in that they have met science-based criteria for safety and effectiveness, but others remain experimental and even questionable, being scientifically groundless and lacking any plausible rationale whatsoever. Some therapies even fit into more than one of these categories depending on the various claims made for them, and the consequent blurring of these distinctions has enabled promoters of quackery and charlatanism to argue that because some practices have merit, the rest deserve equal consideration and respect. This is not, of course, the case, and the large number of spurious and unproven complementary practices are undoubtedly spoiling the territory for those who have much to offer.

Labelling a therapy 'complementary' does not necessarily render it as acceptable as osteopathy or chiropractic, although this is what many would have us believe. Some therapies such as traditional Chinese medicine, have been around for thousands of years; others, such as the Alexander technique, are relatively recent. Some complementary therapists are highly qualified, others have been on a weekend course. Some therapies have set up well-established organizations as regulatory bodies, which have drawn up a code of conduct and provide indemnity in case of errors, others are not regulated at all, and may even be run by a single individual. Some therapists operate as extremely successful businesses, others make a living where they can. It is unfortunate that complementary therapy incorporates so many diverse and contrasting disciplines because the value and worth of one is by no means the equivalent of another.

The Burden of Proof

Under the accepted rules of science, people who make therapeutic claims for any given treatment bear the burden of proof. It remains their responsibility to conduct suitable studies and report them in sufficient detail to permit evaluation and confirmation by others. Conventional medicine does this well. The value of its treatments are believable, because all results and observations are repeatable and verifiable by others. There is a proven consistency and validity which the randomized clinical trial (as described on page 18) is able to demonstrate with unbiased clarity and precision. Such a trial, if it is based on the 'hypothetico-deductive' model described on page 18, can prove irrefutably that a treatment is able to accelerate healing or achieve cure consistently rather than purely by chance. If trials of this sort were taken up by those practising complementary therapy, very few treatments would survive such scrutiny.

Instead of subjecting their work to strict scientific standards, however, promoters of questionable alternative therapies would like to change the rules by which they are judged and regulated. Instead of conducting scientific studies, they use anecdotes and testimonials to promote their practices, and political manoeuvring to keep regulatory agencies at bay. By changing the rules this way, any treatment can be devised which, theoretically, works in every single case. The problem with this is that vulnerable people desperate for an answer to their medical symptoms, but not capable of distinguishing between quackery and science, may be encouraged to spend money on therapies which have no therapeutic value whatsoever.

The Media Bias

The media, which has been so instrumental in destroying much of the population's faith in conventional medicine, has enjoyed a 20-year love affair with complementary therapy. Hundreds of pages of newspapers and magazines are devoted to the subject every week, and television and radio broadcasts that include alternative practices in their output are guaranteed good ratings. Whole departments have been established by the press barons to report on nothing but the latest fad and the most fashionable therapies, and entire squads of non-medically trained journalists compete for column inches. Regrettably, very little critical evaluation is applied to such reports, the articles consisting of thinly disguised 'advertorial' human interest stories of prejudiced testimonials. But the media wields enormous power, and many people still believe all they read in the newspapers. If enough coverage reinforces the notion that complementary therapy is the modern panacea for all ills, growing numbers of the population will eventually believe it. It should not be forgotten, however, that for good moral and ethical reasons, conventionally trained doctors are legally unable to advertise their services in a similar way. The fact that complementary therapists can do this reveals not only that they are not bound by the same strict code of conduct and ethics as the medical fraternity, but also that they can get away with saying what they like about the benefits of their trade.

Too Simple to be True?

Attractive though the philosophies of complementary therapy are, with their focus on the vital life-forces, Chi, miasmas, auras and chakras, simply thinking about health or illness in a different way does not automatically make a treatment any more effective. The understanding of illness in conventional terms is complex, whereas the metaphorical and symbolic notions of energy flow within the body and balanced 'prana' are simple and comprehensible concepts. The trouble is, philosophy on its own cannot cure.

Eccentric and somewhat obsessional reliance on a geomagnetic field or electrophysiological cause of disease can divert people completely from thinking about their health in more useful ways, and such explanations of their disease as 'your aura is weak over your right shoulder' or 'you have an energy blockage in your stomach meridian' are scientifically meaningless and impossible to prove. It is perhaps all very well if a given patient needs to believe that their cure comes from within but, over and above that, it is no more than the diversion of an imaginative mind, attracted to the magical and the mystical, from the stark reality of disease.

Over-Emphasis on Self-Healing

Many complementary therapists are irrepressibly enthusiastic about the concepts of self-healing and the body's capacity to recover from disease from within. No doubt the motivation to give up smoking and cut down on fatty food does come from within; without question the ability of somebody to overcome adversity and prove their capabilities to others is a function of their personality and innate moral fibre. But there are hundreds of thousands of examples of external influences on the body being responsible for infection, cancer, disability and degeneration. How useful is the concept of self-healing in these cases? How damaging is the notion of self-healing for those people born with congenital disease as a result of their genetic make-up? And how appalling it is when complementary therapists advertise their clinics with slogans such as 'CANCER does not choose you – YOU choose cancer'. This implies that when anybody becomes unwell, it is their own fault! It also implies that when they do not get better, they are not trying hard enough to summon up their own inner vital life-source to exorcise the demons of disease. For many, this notion is the last nail in the coffin. It adds insult to injury in the chronically or terminally ill, when the very people who should be supporting them are suggesting that they have shirked their responsibility for staying well. The impact of guilt that they feel and the disappointment they perceive in their so-called healers is just as devastating to such individuals as it is to their friends and families.

The concept of self-healing has other more damaging and potentially lethal implications. When people take it too literally, they are encouraged to abandon all types of conventional therapy, even when it is being prescribed to control serious illness. In the past, such irrational and unshakeable obsession has resulted in lethal consequences. Many a patient undergomg chemotherapy for cancer of the blood, such as leukaemia or lymphoma, have abandoned their treatment in favour of less invasive and pleasanter complementary therapy, only to relapse and die prematurely as a result. In 1994, a situation arose in which four insulin-dependent diabetes sufferers were advised to reduce or curtail their insulin injections and replace them with such alternative practices as faith healing, prayer, exclusion diets and a variety of nutritional supplements. All four suffered weight loss and high blood-sugar levels, and three of them developed the serious condition of ketoacidosis, in which ketones resulting from the unnatural breakdown of fat in the body accumulate in the bloodstream. For one of the three, the condition became life-threatening and permanent damage was caused to the retina at the back of the eye. From this example, it is plain to see that over-reliance on the concept of self-healing as a means of combating organic disease can be extremely hazardous, if not fatal.

The Risks Involved

Despite the cosy image enjoyed by complementary therapy, it also carries risks; injuries, infection, allergic reactions and psychological damage have all been associated with it. Complementary therapy is not subject to the same clinical trials as conventional drugs, and because there is no official reporting system when harmful effects are experienced, few safeguards exist to protect the patient. Moreover, whereas orthodox doctors have to conform to minimum levels of training and qualification, the same is not true of complementary practitioners (some have even been known to give themselves imaginary qualifications by using totally meaningless initials after their name.) However, any good complementary therapist will belong to a professional body which has a code of practice, a complaints system and a disciplinary procedure for when things go wrong, and which insists that all members have professional indemnity insurance.

Herbal preparations have been proven at times to be poisonous, either because the patient has overdosed on the quantity or because contamination with substances such as arsenic and cadmium has taken place. Many products, notably Indian and Chinese medicines, are brought into the country by suppliers with dubious reputations, and are not regulated by any effective law. Physical manipulation techniques used by osteopaths and chiropractors have occasionally damaged the nerves or vertebrae of clients, and even strokes have occassionally been reported. Acupuncturists have been known to damage vital organs, and fragments of broken acupuncture needles have been found in kidneys, spines, hearts, stomachs and livers. The use of acupuncture needles which have not been properly sterilized has also resulted in the transmission of viruses such as hepatitis and HIV. Allergic reactions producing rashes, swelling and stomach problems have been reported from herbal remedies, aromatherapy oils and homeopathic medicines, and may also occur after insertion of metal acupuncture needles. Aromatherapy oils in particular are usually highly concentrated, and must be properly diluted before they are applied to the skin.

Another danger of complementary therapy is that it can influence patients to shun conventional doctors, thus depriving them of the benefits of orthodox treatment. Many homeopaths, for example, oppose immunization and counsel their clients against it. Not only does this expose the patient to the very real dangers of natural disease, but it is also liable to increase the reservoir of contagious illness within the population as a whole, and offset the public health benefits of immunization.

The risks of complementary therapy can be reduced by ensuring you have found a reliable practitioner who is properly qualified and indemnified, and by telling your GP what you are doing. Ascertain exactly what you are taking, if anything, and complain loudly and publicly if you are not fully satisfied with the treatment you are receiveing. Various studies have been carried out to try to measure the degree of risk associated with complementary therapy; some research has reported a complication rate as low as 3 per cent, but others have reported levels as high as 24 per cent. Most of the problems reported have been fairly trivial and short-lived, but there is nevertheless a tangible risk of significant complications, and these should always be borne in mind when complementary therapy is contemplated.

Exaggerated and Misleading Claims

Many complementary therapies are guilty of excessively hyping the benefits of their treatments, but the food supplement industry is amongst the worst. Manufacturers use a wide variety of methods to put across potentially misleading impressions and claims. Not only are many of these claims illegal, but self-regulation by the industry is failing miserably to protect vulnerable consumers. A detailed study by the Food Commission in 1997 found widespread evidence of claims made by the dietary supplement industry which were probably illegal under the UK Medicines Act. Any claims that a product could cure, treat or prevent a disease is a medicinal claim, and any product associated with such a claim requires a medicines licence, but there are dozens of cases of manufacturers making such claims for their products without a licence to do so. Many make carefully worded statements which imply a health benefit, without specifically making any medicinal claim, but the Food Commission found over 700 statements claiming nutritional benefits or overtly medical effects, and felt that existing laws allowed far too much misinterpretation of the rules.

Vitamins, amino acids, enzymes, minerals, fish oils, herbal remedies and dietary supplements marketed as slimming aids were near the top of the list of products for which manufacturers made misleading or illegal claims. The labels on some of these products made claims whilst simultaneously depicting logos and pictures inferring a health benefit, such as a beautiful, smiling fashion model or a picture of a heart. Other products used names which implied a health benefit; e.g. 'immune boost', 'anti-fat' or' 'mobilize'. 'Advertorial's', which are paid-for advertisements/editorials designed to resemble unprejudiced articles in magazines and newspapers, as well as leaflets and books available in-store, support the appeal of these types of goods. So-called independent testimonials are also often used to convince potential customers that if a famous celebrity recovered from, say, cancer by using a certain product, there is no reason why it should not work for them. Of the 741 medicinal claims made by products investigated by the Food Commission in 1997, only 13 held medicines licences. Nearly 100 made claims pertaining to metabolism or digestion, using phrases such as 'alleviating arthritis', 'toning the skin', 'aiding joint mobility' or 'supporting enzyme activity'. Sixty more claimed to be able to aid the cardio-vascular system and suggested they were capable of lowering cholesterol and boosting the immune system. Thirty products made claims relating to weight loss, fat burning and slimming, whilst still more endorsements related to the body's nervous and glandular systems, to reproductive health, eyesight and mental function. Some even claimed to be able to delay the ageing process, and to maintain health whilst travelling. Consumers should be encouraged to ask what evidence there is that olive leaf extract is 'a natural treatment for HIV', and to question whether propolis truly is 'effective in treating hypertension and coronary heart disease', and they should also look carefully at claims made for products such as aloe vera, cat's claw, DHEA (dihydroepiandrosterone) and spirulaena.

Whom Can You Believe?

The UK food labelling regulations expressly forbid labels and advertisements from making any specific or implied claim that a food or food supplement is capable of preventing, treating or curing a human disease. A disease is defined as 'any adverse condition of the body or mind'. The problem with this regulation is that it allows manufacturers to exploit a loophole in that they can still claim that their products help maintain good health, rather than prevent disease. For the consumer, this can be confusing. The label on an iron supplement product, for example, could quite reasonably state that the product contained a given amount of iron. This is a nutrient claim. It could also say that iron is essential to the production of healthy red blood cells. This is a health claim. It could even say that the iron in the product could prevent anaemia. This is a medicinal claim. However, few products can show with any degree of scientific confidence that they are as reliably effective as iron in the maintenance of health and the prevention of disease. Such an iron supplement product would probably have no diffictulty in obtaining a licence as a medicine under the Medicines Control Agency; it would be granted a PL (product licence) number to display on its packaging, and the product would have to undergo tests for safety, quality, standards and effectiveness. It would have to show that it was safe in normal use, with minimal side effects, and that it was capable of achieving what it claimed it could. Regrettably, many disreputable companies get away with using phrases such as 'boosts the immune system', 'burns fat', and 'detoxifies and restores', and with claiming that their product has traditionally been used for a certain condition.

Further confusion arises because, in health food shops and chemists, licensed and unlicensed products containing almost identical ingredients may be positioned side by side on the shelf. All of the above influences the consumers unfairly without offering them any protection. Care needs to be exerted in order to avoid the public being exploited through their relative lack of nutritional expertise. Clearly, the regulations need to be tightened up. The Medicines Control Agency, which is part of the Department of Health, is responsibe for medicinal claims, and the Local Authority Trading Standards Office retains responsibility for controlling misleading claims and labelling. Together with the Advertising Standards Authority, these organizations must pull together more effectively in the future if blatant infringements of the law are to be avoided.

Vulnerable Children

Many parents who are enthusiastic about complementary therapy are happy for their children to receive the same treatment. Herbal remedies, homeopathy and cranial osteopathy, for example, are gentle treatments that carry few side effects and, by and large, are entirely suitable for children. However, certain forms of alternative medicine can put the well-being of children very much at risk, despite the fact that parents have a moral and legal responsibility to protect their health and indeed their lives. In one famous case, a little girl by the name of Lorie Atikian died at the age of 17 months from malnutrition because her parents fervently believed in the power of a peculiar variant of herbalism. Like many complementary therapists, her parents disapproved of conventional medicine and refused to let their daughter be routinely vaccinated against the common and threatening childhood diseases, instead subjecting her to a bizarre cocktail of herbalism and mysticism. Part of the treatment involved wrapping her in cabbage leaves. So strong was her parents' obsession with the treatment and the therapist that they could not see what was happening – that their precious daughter was wasting away and dying before their very eyes. Most reputable complementary therapists would, of course, abhor this type of behaviour, but in one particular branch of spiritual healing, namely that of Christian Science, conventional medicine is specifically forbidden. All illness is regarded as 'discord of the body', and only God is seen as capable of bringing about a cure. Unfortunately, there are several cases where this kind of dogma has led to the death of children. All parents must temper their own strong beliefs and philosophies with a sound medical responsibility for their children.

CHAPTER 6

Integrated Medicine: The Best of Both Worlds

Integrated medicine combines the very best of conventional and alternative medical practices. In doing so, it is able to overcome many of the obvious weaknesses and limitations of both, and hundreds of thousands of patients, who might previously have been denied the help they needed, can obtain the ideal treatment, tailored to their specific requirements. Integrated medicine allows orthodox doctors and alternative practitioners to practise side by side in a non-exclusive partnership in which each can learn from the other and each respects the other's unique contribution and input. There is a pressing and urgent need for therapeutic intervention from both sides, and the overall world of health care would be a much richer and happier place if orthodox and alternative practitioners were able to function synergistically.

Meeting a Very Real Need

Conventionally trained doctors will always be the first port of call for patients suffering from life-threatening and acute conditions, such as insulin-dependent diabetes, severe asthma, epilepsy or meningitis; they will always be the most appropriate experts for patients to turn to with potentially curable but overwhelmingly serious illnesses such as Hodgkin's disease or leukaemia; surgeons who excise diseased organs and transplant healthy ones will always be indispensable. But however well trained and experienced these physicians and surgeons may be, they often remain hopelessly ill-equipped to deal with the 50 per cent of patients who consult them with symptoms that stubbornly defy medical diagnosis, whose complaints are to all intents and purposes minor or trivial, or whose conditions are relapsing and remittent, unproven, chronic or terminal. With all their sophisticated technology, their intensive training and diagnostic acumen, orthodox doctors remain clueless and impotent when it comes to managing those patients whose problems stem from their lifestyle or their emotional and social environment. That many conventionally trained doctors can totally ignore and dismiss the recognized symptoms of severe depression and extreme physical and mental exhaustion in patients merely because they do not believe that ME (myalgic encephalomyelitis) exists, is a case in point. Yet such patients need therapy too, albeit of a different kind. The more tangible and clinically recognized classical diseases as such will always require specific medical attention, but any human being who suffers in any way whatsoever, still needs a little magic to make them well again. Stark clinical facts alone, even when coupled with white coats and stethoscopes, are not sufficient to achieve healing, and there is much that orthodox doctors can learn from their complementary counterparts about becoming better healers who are more effectively equipped to look after the unique and individual human beings in their medical care.

A More Human Approach

A better bedside manner would be one of the first improvements. These days some specialists seem to believe that looking at X-ray films is more important than looking into the patient's eyes, and the doctor–patient relationship seems to have become less important than laboratory analysis. If doctors could only adopt the caring and compassionate approach of many complementary therapists who seem innately skilled in these practices, what an advance for the patient it would be. If tenderness, therapeutic touch, openness, honesty and empathy could all be taken on board, and incorporated into mainstream clinical practice along with so simple and natural a thing as a smile, how much warmer and more rewarding the medical consultation could become. And if communication skills could only parallel diagnostic and investigative ability, how much better informed and how much less apprehensive patients would become. Integrated medicine is capable of making this happen, not only to the benefit of the patient, but also to the doctor and the alternative therapist alike.

Who To Go To First

In the present climate the vast majority of patients consult their orthodox physician first. However, since many orthodox treatments create unwanted side effects and fail to address the underlying cause of the problem, long-term solutions are often not forthcoming. Complementary therapists are usually only consulted when conventional remedies continually fail to come up with satisfactory results. Clearly, there are many situations where this state of affairs should be reversed and, the complementary practitioner would be the ideal person to consult before seeing anyone else. Think of all the benefits of this type of treatment. Firstly, all of those non-specific ailments, like food intolerance, eczema, irritable bowel syndrome and attention deficit hyperactivity disorder, so readily dismissed by many conventional doctors, and all those nebulous, ill-defined and vague problems experienced by half of our population, could finally attract sincere consideration and attention. Secondly, some patients would be able to experience, for the first time ever, that unique sense of empowerment which would give them an awareness and educational insight into the problems from which they suffer. They would be protected from being subjected at the outset to invasive and sometimes unnecessary medical tests. Moreover, because complementary therapies in health care are generally cheaper to provide, the integration of complementary medicines alongside the conventional might potentially contribute to an overall provision of health care in the future which would be financially much more sustainable.

Happier Doctors

If complementary therapy could become more acceptable to the orthodox doctors who feel threatened by it, or to those physicians or surgeons who feel obsessively possessive about their patients, the level of stress and disillusionment, which is obvious within the established medical fraternity, would fall dramatically. Prescribing powerful medication with sometimes hazardous side effects, and subjecting patients to invasive and potentially lethal procedures, carries huge responsibility and the toll this takes in terms of depression, addiction, divorce and even suicide is enormous. Universal access for patients to complementary therapy would reduce demand on doctors' time, and enable more time to be devoted to the severe and acute conditions and the crises and emergencies which always, by definition, command the full attention of orthodox doctors.

Empowerment of Patients

Another justification for complementary therapy being integrated into mainstream practice lies in the principle that illness and disease have a vital role to play in the development of the individual as a person, and of the whole of humanity generally. If people have never evolved adequate coping mechanisms and always react to unfavourable circumstances with anxiety, depression or addiction, or withdraw from society as a means of escape, it is hardly surprising that their difficulties will eventually find expression in physical symptomatology. Complementary therapists broadly agree on the holistic principle that all symptoms are messengers of disease within the body, merely outward signs that the organism is struggling against a lack of balance and harmony within. They see such symptoms and ailments as an opportunity for individual and personal growth, and the therapist's role as that of the educator offering enlightenment, assistance and facilitation, empowering the patient to learn and adapt to their new circumstances with the minimum of discomfort, fear and anxiety.

Body and Soul

Finally, the power of the spiritual elements so essential to many of the complementary therapies should not be underestimated. Contrary to the plight faced by many terminally ill patients cared for by conventional doctors who often 'strive to keep alive' at all costs, those patients treated by complementary therapists often no longer fear suffering or even death itself because they are encouraged to see it in the context of transition, of spiritual connection, of serenity, and possibly even as a step towards reincarnation. In this way patients can be encouraged to regard death as something other than a cruel and intransigent enemy that has to be overcome no matter what.

Avoiding the Victim Culture

Conventional doctors are only just beginning to realize that the definition of health is more than just freedom from disease. According to the World Health Organization, the definition of health is 'not the mere absence of symptoms or infirmities, but a state of physical, psychological, spiritual and social well-being'. It is also the ability to react to all of life's circumstances in a manner that enhances capability, responsibility, independence, spontaneity, fulfilment and happiness. Somebody who is unwell or out of sorts is more than a mere patient to be patronized and disempowered by doctors who see themselves as omnipotent life-savers whose guidance is to be blindly followed. People who seek help from healers of any kind should feel themselves to be much more than helpless victims, there to be rescued by experts and unable to contribute in any way to their own well-being and health. Instead, they should be able to ask as many questions as they wish before making any decision with regard to their medical management, and they should be allowed to make their own choices. Integrated medicine allows this to happen and gives patients the opportunity to make a significant contribution to the healing process. Patients become active partners in their own health care, which gives them independence and autonomy and discourages a passive relationship with the doctor. If patients are allowed to see disease as something which merely happens to them randomly, without them having any responsibility for or connection with it whatsoever, they soon see themselves as victims. This victim consciousness may then encourage society as a whole to become more dependent on others and on state benefits, which further stifles individual autonomy, creativity and initiative.

Benefiting the Patient

Integrated medicine enables patients to select the cream of conventional diagnosis and investigative techniques, or at least as much of them as they wish to exploit, but then also remain empowered to control their own destinies and reactions to ill-health by embracing what alternative medicine has to offer. This can benefit patients in myriad ways. The patient who has had a heart attack caused by his intensely stressful existence might undergo the invasive surgical procedure of a triple coronary bypass graft, only to become a cardiac cripple in the future due to the fear of dropping dead at the least little exertion. Alternatively, when endowed with a positive attitude and a more active approach towards the way he leads his life, with the aid of complementary therapies, he could go on to enjoy the next 30 years feeling much happier and fitter than at any other time of his life. The 30-year-old woman with irritable bowel syndrome, investigated at enormous expense but with no definitive conclusion, could easily become depressed and obsessive about her dietary intake. Alternatively, when reminded that no progressive or serious organic disease had been found, she could be encouraged to find other methods of dealing with her digestive system, over-sensitive as it is to the stresses and strains of today's style of living. Even people who are suffering from cancer, who might otherwise want to turn their faces to the wall and die, can benefit from a system of integrated medicine. If their spirit is soaring and they are at peace with the world so that they can make sense of it all, even at the very last stages of life, they can still benefit from soothing complementary messages and a positive spiritual outlook. They may be able to see, even at this critical impasse, that the healthiest option of all is indeed to die.

Benefiting the Doctor

Morale amongst members of the medical profession has never been lower than it is now. Recruitment of general practitioners in the inner cities is extremely difficult, nursing shortages are rife, and at some medical schools one-third of all graduates leave the medical profession to start other careers within the first two years. The majority of family practitioners recently polled in a trade journal survey confessed that they would not choose to study medicine in the current climate if they had their time again.

In view of this overwhelming disillusionment and low morale, is it any wonder that the health of doctors themselves leaves so much to be desired? It is, of course, a hugely stressful and responsible job. When faced with patients with chronic disease, with people whose symptoms are entirely stress-related, and with people who are facing death from terminal illness, it is easy for doctors to feel helpless and impotent. However much they hate using the phrase, 'I'm afraid there is nothing more I can do for you', they still find themselves saying it time and time again. For these doctors, an integrated medical health care system could provide the shot in the arm they so drastically need.

Supportive complementary therapies would empower patients to cope better with their own problems, and encourage them not to be so dependent on their doctor's advice. Alterations to patients' lifestyles, changes to their diet, nutritional supplementation, physical activity and stress management could all help to divert people away from the doctor's surgery and into the gym, the countryside or the health food shop instead. Doctors could work under less stress, and come to appreciate greater job satisfaction if the doctor–patient relationship revolved around equal team work rather than being the one-sided affair it is now. A good doctor never stops learning; incorporating new concepts, techniques and disciplines into his or her therapeutic armamentarium is highly satisfying for most doctors, and many already carry out various complementary therapies within the context of their NHS surgeries. All of them find this rewarding, effective and fulfilling. It means they are able to offer patients hope and support where previously there was none, and enables them to cut down on the use of potent pharmacological products that they know in their heart of hearts, are not being appropriately prescribed. They are once again able to become true healers, and they become better listeners, better empathists and better carers. Far from being threatened by complementary therapy, the medical profession should increasingly be able to see clearly the benefits for doctors themselves, if only they can keep an open mind. Finally, since the more holistic approach of complementary medicine encourages healers to be aware of the impact of their own health on their patients, orthodox doctors, hopefully, would look after themselves better. The majority are either overweight, smoke too much, work under enormous stress, drink excessively, or take too little exercise. If the General Medical Council sent out that once-again-famous edict 'physician, heal thyself', who knows what positive benefits this might in turn bestow on unsuspecting patients?

Benefiting the Complementary Therapist

Although some complementary therapists are quite content to work with patients who have no medical diagnosis whatsoever, and some specifically seek to do so, most prefer to know which investigations have been carried out and what conclusions have been reached by conventional doctors. No self-respecting, reputable complementary therapist would wish to treat patients with serious and significant illnesses for which much more appropriate and potentially life-saving treatment was available through mainstream medical channels. Most complementary therapists would rather work hand in hand with orthodox doctors than secretively or in spite of them. An integrated approach would encourage communication between all parties to everyone's mutual benefit. The complementary therapist is provided with free and open access to the patient's medical records so that he or she is no longer acting blindly, the orthodox doctor is able to share the burden of care and responsibility for the patient, and lastly, and probably most importantly, the patient no longer needs to feel secretive or guilty about exploring non-conventional forms of therapeutic support. Complementary practitioners would therefore see a wider spectrum of cases, they would gain acceptance and validation from the conventionally trained doctors they worked with, and they would have access to the kind of diagnostic resources currently only available to orthodox doctors like GPs and hospital consultants. Integrated medicine would provide more resources and information for complementary therapists without which complementary therapy will remain less valid and acceptable.

Benefiting Society

Giving people back responsibility for their own health is much more likely to create a healthy society. People who fall victim to disease and place themselves in the hands of so-called medical experts disenfranchise and disempower themselves. Their victim-consciousness allows them to fall prey to passive and pathetic behaviour, they lose all initiative and spiritual energy, and become dependent on anything free that society as a whole is prepared to hand out. When fewer patients feel constrained to pressurize their doctors for quick-fix solutions to their difficulties, such as serial courses of antibiotics, painkillers and tranquillizers, fewer problems will be swept under the carpet, fewer side effects will be experienced and fewer non-specific illnesses will escape a more appropriate and effective long-term remedy.

By empowering people and giving them back the responsibility to guide their own destiny, integrated medicine is much more likely to allow people to stand on their own two feet, and to adopt a positive, healthier attitude throughout their lives. On a universal scale, this bolsters integrity, pride and sovereignty, and generally cements much greater social, emotional and behavioural stability.

Complementary Medicine on the NHS?

The incredible surge in the popularity of complementary therapy bears witness to a crying need for an integrated medical system. Over 4 million people visit the clinics of a growing number of complementary practitioners each year, and spend millions of pounds in the process, but few are doing so to the exclusion of their orthodox doctor. Most people want an integrated health service which is available to all, and many people are actively demanding it. A report published in 1997 was the result of eight months of discussion and consultation between royal colleges, leading researchers, medical schools, health care consumers and representative bodies of complementary medicine. It was entitled *Integrated Healthcare – A Way Forward for the Next Five Years*, and it made 28 specific proposals for further consideration and development, including the introduction of effective systems of self-regulation. It also put forward the suggestion that certain complementary therapies should be available at the expense of the NHS rather than being paid for directly by the patient as is generally the situation at present. The implications of this for the Treasury Department are, of course, enormous, and the Minister for Health at the time, Tessa Jowell, commented that she would be asking her officials to contact the chairmen and chairwomen of the various working groups involved in order to explore the recommendations further. Even the British Medical Association cautiously welcomed the report, at the same time pointing out its controversial nature. Complementary practitioners, in particular, are most excited at the prospect of the costs of such a system falling under the financial umbrella of the NHS. Millions of people use alternative therapy, they would correctly point out, and most have to pay. 'There is no reason why,' as one director of the Society of Homeopathy said at the time, 'if that is the treatment that's best for them, they should not get it free like anything else.'

Born-Again Integrated Medicine

Hippocrates practised a rudimentary form of complementary medicine thousands of years ago. Unfortunately, in subsequent periods of history, his excellent model of holistic health care rather fell by the wayside, but recently things have started to look up again. People are taking more responsibility for their own fitness, and are focusing on leading healthier lifestyles. Education has made people more aware of their own ability to prevent ill-health, and of the importance of good nutrition, adequate exercise and behavioural moderation. Doctors are becoming more likely to suggest a trip to the gym or to supply a diet sheet, than to prescribe a powerful drug or a useless tonic, and hundreds of GPs have broadened their horizons by learning new skills like hypnosis, homeopathy, osteopathy or transcendental meditation. Some qualified doctors even work as spiritual healers too. NHS physiotherapists now practise acupuncture, acupressure and all kinds of physical therapies every day in our hospitals, which are also visited by aromatherapists, reflexologists and yoga teachers. Used alongside conventional therapy, complementary treatment is already available in many areas, though its distribution under the NHS remains patchy. Five homeopathic hospitals already exist in the NHS and many fundholding partnerships are able to refer their patients to a variety of complementary therapists working either within the confines of their own premises, or just a short distance away. In doing so, the interdisciplinary co-operation needed to achieve this ensures effective and safe delivery of care.

Models of Integrated Health Care

One model of integrated medicine pioneered by Professor Patrick Pietroni at the Marylebone Health Centre in Central London is a marvellous example of how beautifully the system could work. This large group practice employed a number of conventionally trained GPs and alternatively trained complementary therapists at the Health Centre, which was, and remains, under the remit of the NHS. Not only were doctors and therapists alike delighted to work in such an environment, but patients, too, were thrilled to be offered such a wide range of therapeutic interventions. Amazingly, the drug prescribing rate at the Centre fell to 60 per cent below the national average for ordinary GP surgeries, and to 36 per cent below the local London level. This represented a saving of many thousands of pounds, which offset the cost of the complementary practices. Not only that, but fewer referrals to local consultant specialists had to be made because much of the work could be carried out by the Centre's own acupuncturist or spiritual healer. Furthermore, less call was made upon local psychiatric services because the Centre boasted a counselling and healing service of its own.

Other large group practices within the NHS have set up similar models of integrated health care, albeit on a smaller scale as they are constrained to work within financial budgets dictated by various health authorities and regulatory bodies. However, the general tone and mood is very much to encourage patients to enjoy the best of all medical worlds wherever practicable.

In conventional hospitals, too, complementary therapy truly *complements* orthodox medicine. In the Intensive Care Unit of the Royal Infirmary in Liverpool, patients have the opportunity to experience aromatherapy, carried out by several of the nurses who have trained in various skills and massage techniques with which they can treat patients on a daily basis. Dr Chris Wilkes, who introduced the treatment, said 'Who cares if all we're doing is putting the human contact back into nursing practice on the ICU?' Provided the patients enjoy it and derive benefit from it, it increasingly has a place. Dr Peter Whorwell, Director of Medicine at the Withington Hospital has had fantastic success with irritable bowel syndrome patients through the use of hypnosis, and regularly uses this therapy when other methods of treatment are inappropriate or ineffective. All over the country, there are other examples of specialists who have taken on board the fact that less conventional methods of treatment can benefit their patients, and increasingly an integrated medical approach is being adopted. This ground swell of change would occur very much faster but for the fact that resources are limited and those who control the government's purse strings have yet to be convinced that tax payers' money is well spent in this direction.

But Who is Responsible for the Patient?

In an integrated system of health care, the role of the family doctor is probably of even greater importance. With so much more choice and information available, patients need reassurance and guidance from a single health care professional who can oversee their treatment. This should be someone who knows them well as individuals, who is familiar with their medical records and every aspect of their lives, who is aware of their domestic circumstances and situation, and who is also in contact with all the various specialist practitioners, can give unbiased advice, and has no pecuniary interest in the patient. Retaining his duty of care to the patient from the cradle to the grave, the GP is better trained and suited to the role of 'gatekeeper' in primary health care than any complementary practitioner, and one of the basic strengths of general practice is the multidisciplinary partnership which that entails. At the end of the day, some individual has to retain overall responsibility for the patient. This fact is recognized at the Marylebone Health Centre where GPs always assess patients first before they are referred to the appropriate complementary therapist.

Professional Responsibility

The General Medical Council sets down a code of conduct and defines the medical duties of a doctor, and orthodox practitioners are obliged to abide by this. Some professional bodies of complementary therapies have attempted to do the same, but as yet these are few and far between. Certainly the level of regulation of the various complementary practitioners is patchy and less well defined. In days gone by, it was actually illegal for a conventionally trained doctor to refer any patient to a complementary therapist, but now the GMC recognizes that a doctor may delegate treatment or other procedures to a complementary therapist if it is considered appropriate, but the doctor must be satisfied that the person to whom they are referring the patient is competent enough to carry out such treatment. The GMC also maintains that it is important for the doctor to retain ultimate responsibility for the management of these patients, because only the doctor has received the necessary training. More recently, in 1995, guidelines for the employment of complementary therapists within the NHS were drawn up, and these insist that all such therapists be appropriately qualified, registered and professionally insured. Should anything go wrong, the NHS complaints procedures can be utilized, provided the patient has been seen by the complementary practitioner as an NHS patient. If this is not the case, it is the practitioner who should be approached about the complaint, and if no satisfaction can be had, the professional body to which the therapist belongs, or even an umbrella organization such as the British Complementary Medicine Association or the Institute for Complementary Medicine, might be able to help.

The Future

The future for an integrated system of health care is bright. The public want it, it is already growing rapidly, and cost-effective models established throughout the country have proved its worth. Much more needs to change, however, before a truly comprehensive system of health care that involves all of the different methods of treatment, and which is available to everyone, can be established. As Britain's heir to the throne correctly says, 'It remains an achievable goal which we cannot afford to miss.

PART TWO

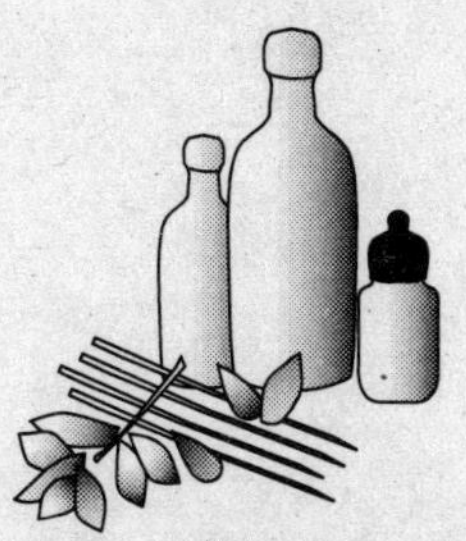

The Alternative Choice

CHAPTER 7

Choosing the Right Complementary Therapy

One of the main principles of complementary therapy is that the treatment must always be specifically tailored to the individual patient's needs. However, with so many different and contrasting therapies to choose from, how does the uninitiated client come to an appropriate decision? Furthermore, since few complementary therapists are likely to admit their limitations in dealing with a particular problem, and refer the potential patient on to someone else, how can the consumer ensure they are seeing the best therapist for the job?

Many patients are motivated to consult a complementary practitioner because orthodox doctors have investigated them and failed to come to any satisfactory conclusion, perhaps because their symptoms are non-specific and nebulous. What form of treatment would be best utilized in this situation? Sometimes the 'consumer', 'client' or 'patient', or however they like to see themselves in any given health situation, will have learned about a particular type of treatment which they feel intuitively would suit them well; it seems to fit in nicely with their outlook and philosophy on life. Others will have been recommended to a specific therapist by a friend, work colleague or relation. Sometimes GPs or other NHS health care workers are open-minded enough to suggest a treatment to them, or even offer to carry out these procedures themselves if they have already undergone the additional training

As we have seen, the family doctor in fact already acts as a kind of 'gatekeeper' for patients who have symptoms that are best treated by conventional methods of health care, and as a result of the multidisciplinary co-operation established between the GP and his health care co-workers in any given area, he or she is also expertly placed to guide any would-be complementary therapy user along the correct path. The GP can use his or her own influence to suggest particular therapists and specific treatments and even possibly to obtain such services free of private charge on the NHS.

It is not essential, of course, nor for that matter usual, for referrals to complementary practitioners to come from family doctors at the present time, but the GP does at least provide a framework for helping patients to select the right treatment if they wish to seek alternative help in attempting to alleviate their symptoms. To some extent, this can protect them from wasting time and money. Complementary health care clinics can themselves provide a similar service but, of course, will have a pecuniary interest in referring customers to one of their own therapists. That said, many such clinics would never dream of suggesting any treatment for a patient that was not wholly appropriate, safe or ethical. Most complementary therapists that I, personally, work with will only take on a patient when they are confident that therapeutic benefit can be obtained.

There are, however, number of pointers that *can* help potential clients select the right therapist:

- Choose a form of treatment with which you feel broadly comfortable and can believe in.
- Find a clinic with a good reputation and track record, or contact one of the professional registers or governing bodies which can supply the name and address of a local practitioner.
- Verify the chosen practitioner's training and membership of an appropriate professional organization.
- Have a good look round the practitioner's premises and assess the attitude of their staff, the atmosphere and the overall level of hygiene and equipment.
- At the first interview, ask the therapist directly if he or she has much experience in treating the condition you are suffering from, and whether they believe they can help.
- Ask for a thorough explanation of the treatment proposed, what it involves, how many sessions will be required, and what the final cost is likely to be.

- Ask the practitioner if he or she will liaise with your family doctor and whether any alteration in the medication you are already taking will be necessary.

By and large, if most people follow these simple steps before embarking on a new form of complementary therapy, they will not be exploited or disappointed. Remember that personal recommendation from a friend is not sufficient in itself; people have different symptoms, different attitudes to ill-health, and react differently towards healers and treatments, so the fact that your neighbour attributes a miracle cure to the local iridologist does not mean that your own irritable bowel syndrome will dramatically disappear if you see him or her as well.

Another major factor in determining the right kind of complementary therapy for you is the nature of your condition. Clearly, very acute organic diseases, such as appendicitis, perforated peptic ulcer and epileptic convulsions, are never going to be suitable for treatment by complementary therapists. Perhaps prevention of these conditions might be, but their immediate treatment once they have developed never can be. More chronic, relapsing, less specific symptoms, however, may certainly fall squarely under the therapeutic umbrella of many of the complementary therapies. Iatrogenic disorders, that is those conditions brought about by the actions and treatments of orthodox doctors themselves, are also suitable for alternative medical treatments, and so are all of the numerous stress-related conditions which affect so many of our overwrought, hyperactive and exhausted population.

As a rough guide, it is reasonable to suggest that certain complementary therapies are better first choices than others in attempting to solve particular medical conditions. Hypnotherapy for example is an excellent first choice for someone suffering from a social phobia; aromatherapy, on the other hand, would tend to be less effective in this individual situation. Similarly, chiropractic would be better for certain types of back pain than herbal medicine; nutritional therapy better than massage therapy for premenstrual syndrome, and so on. The following table is an attempt to offer readers a basic guide to which complementary treatment might be most useful for a large number of common system-

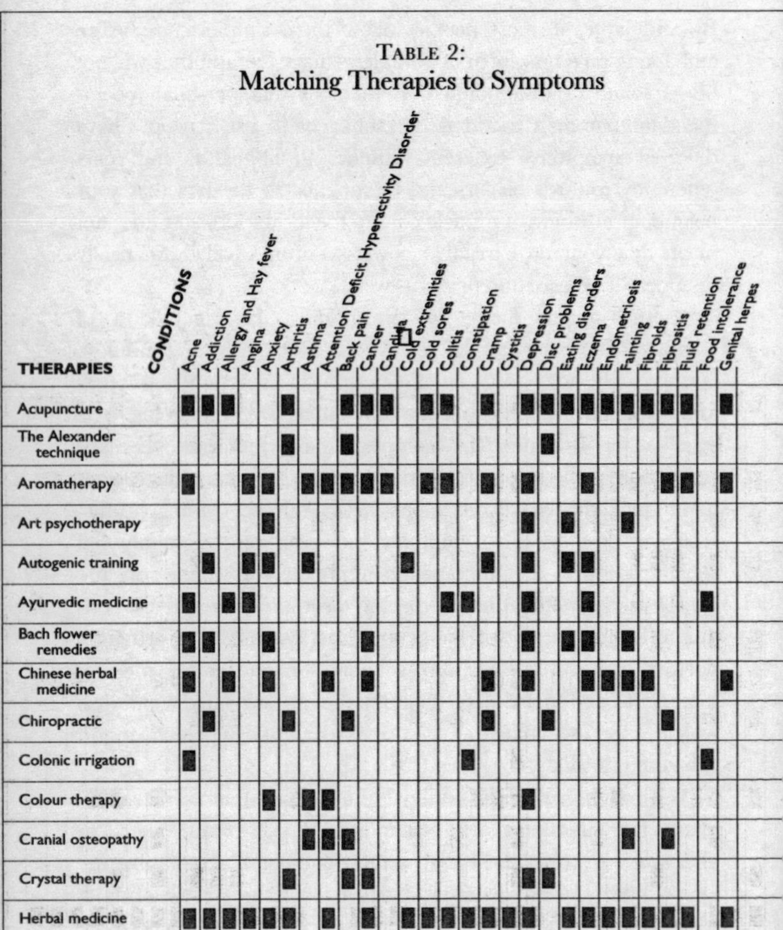

TABLE 2:
Matching Therapies to Symptoms

THERAPIES / CONDITIONS	Acne	Addiction	Allergy and Hay fever	Angina	Anxiety	Arthritis	Asthma	Attention Deficit Hyperactivity Disorder	Back pain	Cancer	Candida	Cold extremities	Cold sores	Colitis	Constipation	Cramp	Cystitis	Depression	Disc problems	Eating disorders	Eczema	Endometriosis	Fainting	Fibroids	Fibrositis	Fluid retention	Food intolerance	Genital herpes
Acupuncture	■	■	■			■			■	■	■		■	■		■		■	■	■	■	■	■	■	■	■		■
The Alexander technique						■			■										■									
Aromatherapy	■			■	■		■	■	■	■	■		■	■		■		■			■				■	■		■
Art psychotherapy					■													■		■			■					
Autogenic training		■		■	■		■					■				■		■		■	■							
Ayurvedic medicine	■		■	■										■	■			■			■						■	
Bach flower remedies	■	■			■					■								■		■	■		■					
Chinese herbal medicine	■		■		■			■		■						■		■			■	■	■	■				■
Chiropractic		■				■			■							■			■						■			
Colonic irrigation	■														■												■	
Colour therapy					■		■	■										■										
Cranial osteopathy							■	■	■														■		■			
Crystal therapy						■			■	■								■	■									
Herbal medicine	■	■	■	■	■	■		■		■		■	■	■	■	■	■	■		■	■	■	■	■	■	■		■

related disorders. There will, of course, be a considerable degree of overlap in the therapeutic ranges of various treatments, and more than one therapy could feasibly be experienced simultaneously.

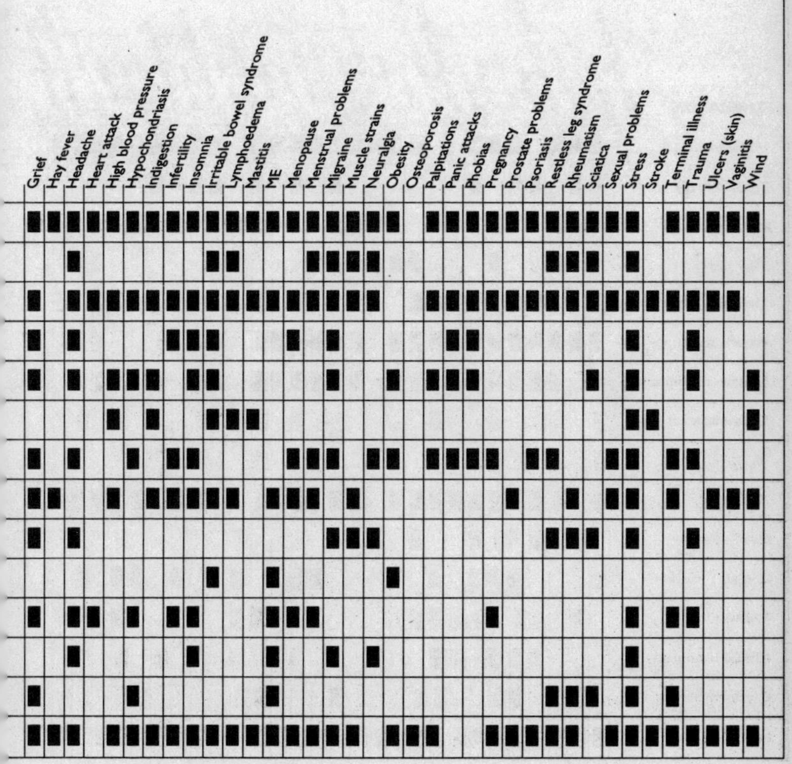

TABLE 2: Matching Therapies to Symptoms

Grief	Hay fever	Headache	Heart attack	High blood pressure	Hypochondriasis	Indigestion	Infertility	Insomnia	Irritable bowel syndrome	Lymphoedema	Mastitis	ME	Menopause	Menstrual problems	Migraine	Muscle strains	Neuralgia	Obesity	Osteoporosis	Palpitations	Panic attacks	Phobias	Pregnancy	Prostate problems	Psoriasis	Restless leg syndrome	Rheumatism	Sciatica	Sexual problems	Stress	Stroke	Terminal illness	Trauma	Ulcers (skin)	Vaginitis	Wind
■	■	■	■	■	■	■	■	■	■	■	■	■	■	■	■	■	■	■		■	■	■	■	■	■	■	■	■	■	■		■	■	■	■	■
		■							■	■				■	■	■	■									■	■	■		■						
■		■	■	■	■	■	■	■	■	■	■	■	■	■	■	■	■			■	■	■	■	■	■	■	■	■	■	■	■	■	■	■	■	
■		■					■	■	■				■		■						■	■								■			■			
■		■		■	■	■		■	■						■			■		■	■	■						■		■			■			■
				■		■			■	■	■																			■	■					■
■		■			■		■	■					■	■	■		■	■		■	■	■	■		■	■			■	■		■	■			
■	■			■		■	■	■	■	■		■	■	■		■								■			■		■	■		■		■	■	■
■		■													■	■	■									■	■	■		■			■			
									■			■						■																		
■		■	■		■		■	■				■	■	■									■							■		■	■			
		■						■				■			■		■													■						
■					■							■														■	■	■		■		■				
■	■	■		■	■	■	■	■	■	■	■	■	■	■	■	■		■	■	■			■	■	■	■	■		■	■	■	■	■	■	■	■

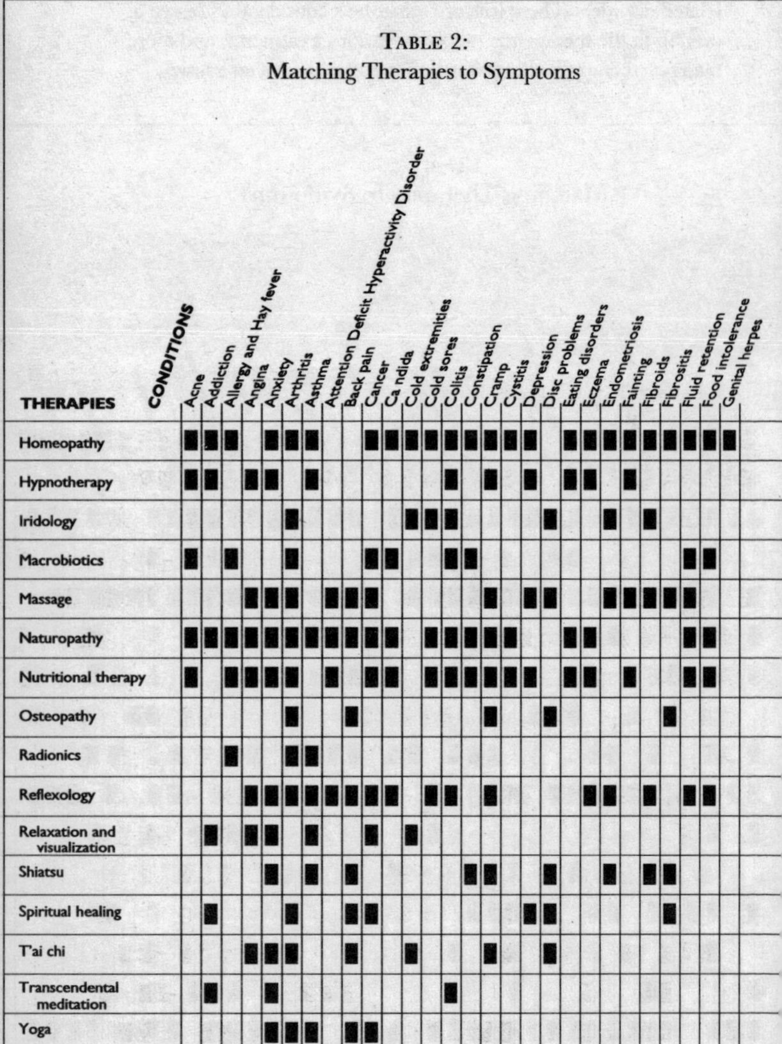

TABLE 2:
Matching Therapies to Symptoms

THERAPIES / CONDITIONS	Acne	Addiction	Allergy and Hay fever	Angina	Anxiety	Arthritis	Asthma	Attention Deficit Hyperactivity Disorder	Back pain	Cancer	Ca ndida	Cold extremities	Cold sores	Colitis	Constipation	Cramp	Cystitis	Depression	Disc problems	Eating disorders	Eczema	Endometriosis	Fainting	Fibroids	Fibrositis	Fluid retention	Food intolerance	Genital herpes
Homeopathy	■	■	■		■	■	■			■	■	■	■	■	■	■	■	■		■	■	■	■	■	■	■	■	■
Hypnotherapy	■	■		■	■		■							■		■		■		■	■		■					
Iridology						■						■	■	■					■			■		■				
Macrobiotics	■		■			■				■	■			■	■											■	■	
Massage				■	■	■		■	■	■						■		■	■			■	■	■	■	■		
Naturopathy	■	■	■	■	■	■	■	■	■	■	■		■	■	■	■	■			■	■					■	■	
Nutritional therapy	■		■	■	■	■		■		■	■		■	■	■	■	■	■		■	■		■			■	■	
Osteopathy						■			■							■			■						■			
Radionics			■			■	■																					
Reflexology				■	■	■	■	■	■	■	■		■	■		■					■	■		■		■	■	
Relaxation and visualization		■		■	■		■			■		■																
Shiatsu					■		■		■						■	■			■			■		■	■			
Spiritual healing		■				■			■	■								■	■						■			
T'ai chi				■	■	■			■			■				■			■									
Transcendental meditation		■			■									■														
Yoga					■	■	■		■	■																		

TABLE 2:
Matching Therapies to Symptoms

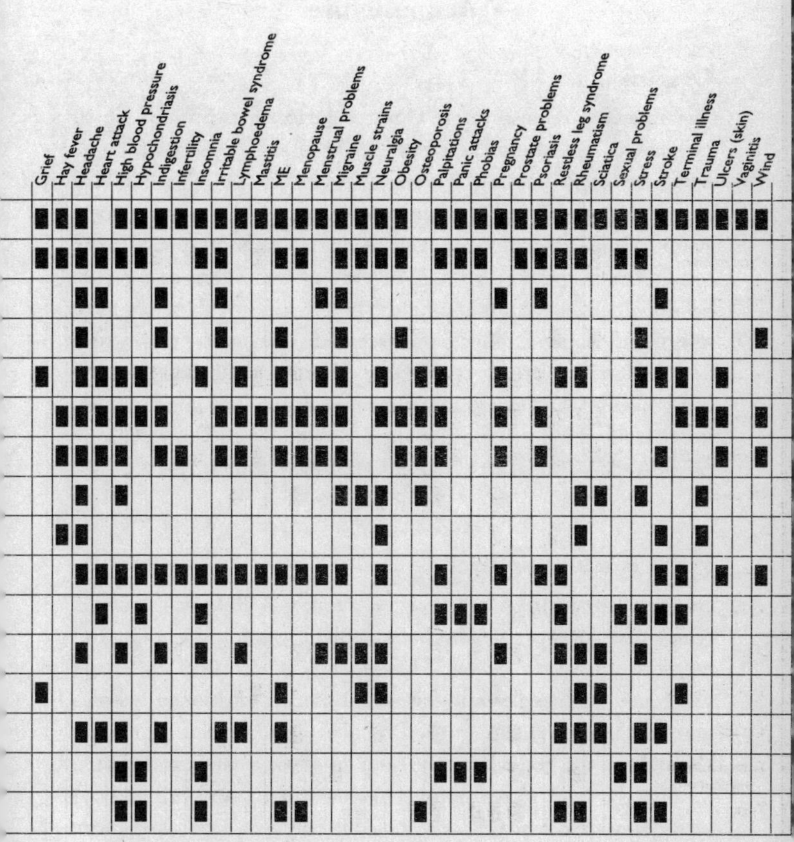

Grief	Hay fever	Headache	Heart attack	High blood pressure	Hypochondriasis	Indigestion	Infertility	Insomnia	Irritable bowel syndrome	Lymphoedema	Mastitis	ME	Menopause	Menstrual problems	Migraine	Muscle strains	Neuralgia	Obesity	Osteoporosis	Palpitations	Panic attacks	Phobias	Pregnancy	Prostate problems	Psoriasis	Restless leg syndrome	Rheumatism	Sciatica	Sexual problems	Stress	Stroke	Terminal illness	Trauma	Ulcers (skin)	Vaginitis	Wind
■	■	■		■	■	■	■	■	■	■	■	■	■	■	■	■	■	■		■	■	■	■	■	■	■	■	■	■	■	■	■	■	■	■	■
■	■	■	■	■	■			■	■			■	■		■	■	■	■		■	■	■		■	■	■	■		■	■						
		■	■			■			■					■	■								■		■						■					
		■				■			■			■			■			■												■						■
■		■	■	■	■			■		■		■		■	■		■		■	■			■			■	■			■	■	■		■		
	■	■	■	■	■	■			■	■	■	■	■	■	■		■	■	■	■			■		■							■	■	■		■
	■	■	■	■		■	■		■	■		■	■	■	■			■	■	■			■		■						■			■		■
		■		■											■	■	■		■								■	■		■			■			
	■	■															■										■				■		■			
		■	■	■	■	■	■	■	■	■	■	■	■	■	■		■			■			■		■	■					■	■		■		■
			■		■			■												■	■	■				■			■	■	■	■				
		■		■		■		■		■				■	■	■	■						■			■	■	■		■						
■												■				■	■										■	■				■				
		■	■	■		■			■	■		■														■	■	■		■	■					
				■	■			■												■	■	■							■	■		■				
				■	■			■				■	■						■							■	■			■	■					

CHAPTER 8

An A–Z of Complementary Therapies

Acupuncture

Origins

Acupuncture is an ancient Chinese form of treatment which originated anywhere between 2,000 and 5,000 years ago. Folklore suggests that it was developed by the medical practitioners of that era who reported that soldiers wounded in battle by piercing objects, such as arrowheads or spears, were sometimes miraculously cured of chronic conditions or injuries. By documenting and mapping the precise sites of these wounds, and the therapeutic effects they seemed to promote, these early acupuncturists were then able to experiment with skin piercing using needles, and eventually drew up a manual of acupuncture, the first of which was entitled the *Huang-di Nei-jing* (Inner Classic of the Yellow Emperor). This was published around 200 BC.

What is acupuncture?

Acupuncture forms a large part of traditional Chinese medicine, which also incorporates herbalism, dietary therapy, t'ai chi and moxibustion (see below). Essentially, it involves inserting extremely fine needles into the skin at specific locations known as acupoints, which can be used to alter the balance of energy throughout the body. It can be both a holistic treatment designed to alter the body's own natural healing energy and bring about well-being, good health and long life, or it can be used more specifically, as in 'Western' or 'scientific' acupunture to treat particular complaints, such as pain, arthritis or insomnia.

How does it work?

The philosophy of ancient Chinese medicine is complex, but if you really want to know more about how acupuncture works in the holistic sense, you need to be familiar with the basics. It is certainly worth familiarizing yourself with the few commonly used 'buzz' words which will crop up should you ever decide to see an acupuncturist and listen to the explanation they are likely to give you. The laws of the Dao or Tao philosophy broadly deal with life-style and behaviour, and they are designed to encourage moderation, harmony and balance in all things. The reasoning is that we are all driven by three 'treasures', Chi or Qi (pronounced 'chee'), Shen and Jing. The treasure Chi equates to energy, Shen to the spirit and Jing to the soul, or being.

A traditional acupuncturist's job is to improve someone's health by helping them to abide more closely to the laws of the Dao, which means avoiding an existence of excess and extreme. Working too hard, drinking too much, over-anxiety or promiscuity would all therefore by frowned upon. They would be regarded as permanently depleting your Jing, and as a consequence affecting your personal growth, self-esteem and development.

Another essential idea within Chinese thought is the importance of balancing the opposing forces of Yin and Yang. Illness is regarded as the consequence of these two elements being in disharmony and disequilibrium, and the acupuncturist's aim is to restore this. Yin is feminine, cold, dark and passive, whereas Yang is the opposite – masculine, warm, light and active. Nothing is ever entirely one or the other; Yin and Yang always interrelate and only when they combined together are they liable to make up the whole. It is when one becomes a dominant force at the expense of the other that illness or unhappiness may be the result.

The Yin and Yang philosophy is further developed into the system of five elements, namely wood, fire, earth, metal and water, all of which are seen to possess certain associations with our physical, emotional and spiritual health. If this seems rather nebulous and vague, by way of example, someone who is deemed to have an imbalance in their fire element may be red or flushed in the face, may be jovial and ebullient, might crave bitter-tasting foods, love hot weather and be prone to heart or circulatory problems. In this kind of way, 'five-element diagnosis' is used to identify areas of disharmony in a patient's life so that treatment can then be administered to restore equilibrium to the body, mind and spirit.

Like many of the other complementary therapies based on a vitalistic philosophy of 'life-force' or 'vital energy', acupuncture is founded on the simple concept of Chi. Chi represents an invisible flow of energy around the body channelled through 12 'meridians' or pathways, six of which are Yin, and six are Yang. Each meridian is named after an anatomical organ or function of the body, and there are 365 major acupuncture points scattered along them.

The basic tenet is that when Chi courses fluently through the meridians, the body is balanced and healthy, but when the energy flow becomes disturbed, diminished or blocked, physical, psychological or emotional disorders can occur. In this way, it is understood that unresolved emotional conflict, which results in anger, depression or anxiety, can eventually lead to organic, physical illness. To correct such imbalances an acupuncturist might take a two-way approach, advising his or her client to make adjustments to their everyday life, while also attempting to correct any imbalances in the patient's Chi, Shen or Jing by using the acupoints. This might, for example, mean advising the client about a better diet and reducing their level of exercise or stress as well as inserting acupuncture needles into specific points to either stimulate or inhibit energy flow.

Conventionally trained users of acupuncture believe that it works within the nervous system by releasing substances which are naturally produced opiate painkillers, and which have a powerful effect on the sensation of pain. These are the same endorphins or 'happy' hormones that are enhanced after regular exercise or excitement, and may be the reason why people do not feel the pain of even a severe injury when it is incurred in the heat of battle or on the playing field. Another explanation is that acupuncture works along the lines of the 'gate' theory, which states that there are physiological gates along the spinal cord which can open or close to let pain through, or not, as the case may be. The gates can be controlled by blocking the transmission of severe pain along nerve fibres by stimulating other nerve fibres with gentle tactile applications, such as acupuncture or acupressure. The gate theory is thought to explain how a mother rubbing her sick child's sore tummy can somehow make the pain easier.

Is acupuncture effective?

Unlike many other complementary therapies which have yet to satisfactorily demonstrate, in any meaningful scientific way, that they work, acupuncture has now merited enough credibility to be widely accepted by the orthodox medical establishment. This is so much the case that acupuncture is now practised throughout the Western world and in particular within state-run NHS hospitals and GP clinics. A great many state-registered physiotherapists and GPs have been impressed enough by the efficacy of acupuncture to have learned the skills and incorporated them into their mainstream clinical practices.

Acupuncture certainly makes people feel better, and several hundred randomized trials have suggested that it truly helps relieve symptoms. One study showed that patients with osteoarthritis experienced a significant reduction in knee pain after acupuncture. A number of them even benefited so much that they actually cancelled the surgical operations they had already consented to, and were therefore able to avoid all the psychological trauma and anaesthetic risks that attend them.

Other research suggests that the treatment can abolish some of the nausea and discomfort associated with chemotherapy, childbirth and surgery, and some work has also implied that acupuncture might even be of use in respiratory conditions like asthma. A study published in the *Lancet* in 1989 highlighted the value of acupuncture in treating chronic alcoholics (it reduced the number of drinking bouts they had and their re-admissions to detoxification units), and more recent work has confirmed this simple therapy can assist other addicts, notably those dependent on crack and cocaine. The jury is still out on whether acupuncture significantly helps people stop smoking, but anything which brings addicts into contact with therapists in an attempt to kick a bad habit must surely have some intrinsic value of its own.

Even patients suffering from the chest pain of angina can experience an improvement in their symptoms by using acupuncture. A small Swedish study showed that patients with coronary heart disease suffered less frequent episodes of pain even though their cardiac performance on exercise testing showed no change.

It is likely, in view of this growing scientific evidence, that the use of acupuncture will continue to spread and be increasingly incorporated into conventional clinical practice. Apart from anything else, the more subjective improvement in patients' general well-being in the face of a wide variety of medical complaints makes acupuncture an extremely valuable weapon in the therapist's armamentarium of treatments.

What form might the treatment take?

Just as conventional doctors cannot correctly start treating a patient until a definitive diagnosis has been made, so acupuncturists also begin by forming a diagnosis. The patient will be asked about their lifestyle and their symptoms and also what particularly has brought them for treatment. At the same time, the therapist will observe things in the patient, such as their complexion, the lustre of their eyes and any coating on their tongue. Touching the patient's skin to feel for hot or cold areas, and a unique form of pulse-taking, will almost certainly also be practised. In traditional Chinese acupuncture there are six pulses, three at each wrist, and there are 28 descriptions of pulse quality, which are used as a guide to diagnosis. Unlike the pulse qualities described by orthodox doctors who might use terms like 'rapid', 'shallow', 'bounding' or 'collapsing', traditional Chinese acupuncturists match the six various pulses to those described in ancient texts and might record their nature somewhat symbolically as 'spring water welling up', 'multiple as the seeds of the flower blossom' or simply 'choppy' or 'slippery'.

Once a diagnosis has been reached using these and other related methods, the acupuncturist will decide on a plan of action to restore the energy balance in the patient's body. The therapist will then insert fine stainless steel needles into the acupoints that have been selected, usually using anything from two to eight needles in all. Depending on the site chosen and the depth to which the needles are inserted, there may be a slight pricking sensation or a diffuse ache, but the discomfort is mild and unobtrusive, and is nothing at all like the rather nauseating discomfort that patients sometimes experience when orthodox doctors use the wider bore needles to take blood samples. This is the basic technique of 'needling'. The amount of time the acupuncture needles may be left in the skin varies, from a couple of seconds to anything up to 45 minutes. Finally, based on whether the acupuncturist feels that each acupoint needs stimulating or calming, a variety of techniques may be employed to correct the required energy flow around the body.

Moxibustion

Moxibustion, a small cone of powdered moxa, a drug derived from the dried herb lugwort, is applied to an acupoint, either at the top of an acupuncture needle or directly on the acupoint itself. The moxa is ignited, giving off not only a pleasant aromatic smell but also sending warmth and stimulating energy through to the acupoint beneath. This technique is designed to warm and stimulate the Qi.

Cupping

This technique uses special cups, made from a variety of material such as glass or wood which are placed over the skin and warmed in order to create a vacuum which will draw the skin into it. This is another way of encouraging blood flow and energy to the acupoint beneath and its surrounding area. Obviously this can only be used on flat areas of the body such as the back or chest.

Electro-acupuncture

This technique is a much more recent variation on traditional acupuncture, and involves the use of a small electrical current to stimulate the acupoints. This type of acupuncture is the basis of the TENS machine, the Trans-cutaneous Electrical Nerve Stimulator, which is commonly used these days for the control of pain during childbirth.

Laser acupuncture

Laser acupuncture is sometimes given to toddlers and children, or for that matter to adults who may be wary or afraid of needles. The laser beam merely represents another form of energy which again can be used on particular acupoints, but it has the advantage of causing very little, if any sensation in the skin.

What problems are helped by acupuncture?

According to the philosophy of ancient traditional Chinese acupuncture, this therapy can promote a long and healthy life and enhance general well-being. It is therefore used for a wide variety of complaints and ailments, and seems to be particularly well received in those patients who feel generally out of sorts and tired all the time. Acupuncture is increasingly being recognized by conventional medical doctors as a very useful adjunct to pain relief in a host of clinical situations. It is particularly useful during childbirth; unlike other remedies, it cannot do any harm to the baby, and is thought to be able to reduce the pain of childbirth by up to one-third.

Acupuncture is also very useful for treating arthritis and muscle pain, and it has been adopted in many NHS pain clinics around the country, where it enables patients to reduce their dose of more conventional drugs, and consequently suffer less side effects as a result of them. It is even used in patients with cancer to reduce the nausea and vomiting they experience after chemotherapy.

Acupuncture also seems to reduce withdrawal symptoms for people coming off hard drugs such as heroin and cocaine, although it is more commonly used to help people stop smoking or drinking excessively. The applications of the principles of traditional acupuncture mean that it can be used for an enormous range of emotional, physical and psychological problems, and it is therefore used in the relief of migraine, menopause, menstrual problems, high blood pressure, insomnia, depression, stress and anxiety, sinusitis, hay fever, digestive problems such as irritable bowel syndrome, and many other common ailments where stress may be an underlying factor.

Quite apart from reducing nausea resulting from orthodox treatment for terminal illness, acupuncture may also help patients to find an inner calmness of spirit and emotional control with which to deal with the difficult path ahead.

Is it safe?

Acupuncture uses sterile stainless steel needles that are incredibly thin, so it is easy to assume that they cannot do any harm. It is true that they are usually only 1–2.5cm (½– 1 inch) long, and are only inserted into the skin to a depth of up to 5mm (¼ inch) but there are a number of problems that can be associated with acupuncture. A Norwegian study published in 1996 documented problems including local skin infections, fainting during the procedure and even pneumothorax (punctured lung) as a result of excessively deep needle insertion, probably in the area just above the clavicle where the apex of the lung is quite superficial to the skin. Unsterilized needles can also transmit serious and life-threatening infections such as hepatitis and the AIDS virus, just as the needles in tattooing can. It is vital therefore that a fully qualified practitioner, who will use sterile disposable needles, is chosen. With these provisos in mind, acupuncture should be perfectly safe for everybody. Whilst even young children and pregnant women can undergo therapy, all the precautions which are usually taken by practitioners of orthodox medicine when treating these groups should still apply.

Finally, it is worth saying that, occasionally, an increase rather than a decrease in the level of pain occurs after treatment. Therapists believe this is a positive sign indicating that physical, mental and emotional problems are being brought to the surface. In these situations, they advise continuing with treatment in the anticipation of future improvement.

How can I find an acupuncturist?

Although the incidence of serious complications resulting from acupuncture worldwide numbers only about 200 over a 20-year period, the business of inserting needles beneath people's skin should never be undertaken lightly. It is imperative therefore to check the qualifications of a potential acupuncturist, especially as, at the present, there is absolutely nothing to stop anybody setting themselves up as an acupuncturist with no training or experience whatsoever. Depending on the type of acupuncture you require, traditional Chinese or Western scientific, you can find suitably trained and registered practitioners either via the British Acupuncture Council (BAC) or the British Medical Acupuncture Society (BMAS).

Medical acupuncture is carried out by conventionally trained medical practitioners who have had additional training in acupuncture and use the treatment as an extension to their more orthodox skills. It may well be that your own NHS GP is registered with the BMAS as there are now over 1,400 doctors in the Society. There are a similar number of therapists on the register of the BAC and many of these work in conjunction with GPs, either on the same premises or a short distance from them. My advice is to make sure the therapist you have in mind is fully registered with a governing body which adheres to a code of conduct and ethics, and that the therapist is covered by some kind of liability insurance. Ask before you begin how much the treatment will cost and how many appointments and consultations you are likely to need.

How much will it cost?

The cost of acupuncture obviously varies from therapist to therapist, and often depends on the area in which he or she practises. If any additional herbs or pills are prescribed, these will obviously need to be paid for as well. By and large the cost of each appointment will be somewhere between £20 and £40.

The sceptic's view

The sceptic, whilst grudgingly accepting that there is a small place for acupuncture in mild to moderate pain relief in conventional clinical practice, would still find the philosophy of traditional Chinese acupuncture fanciful and far-fetched. He or she would point out that the relatively small number of randomized trials on the efficacy of the therapy are not wholly conclusive, and that those studies which cast doubt on its use for helping smokers give up the habit show it to be no more successful than the use of nicotine chewing gum. The sceptic would find the claim that stimulating a special acupoint located on the little toe can help to turn an unborn baby in a breach position in the mother's womb to a head-down position particularly laughable. Disbelievers have made much of the fact that, even in China, acupuncture alone is never used in surgery, especially emergency surgery, and that no scientific evidence can confirm the so-called flow of energy along invisible meridians. Lastly, and perhaps most importantly, the sceptic would feel that the patient runs a real risk of the non-medically-qualified acupuncturist missing a vital diagnosis of serious disease. It is all very well pandering to the patient's need for spiritual uplifting and mysticism, but not if it means a potentially curable abdominal tumour, early-stage blood cancer, or heart valve defect is totally missed.

The therapist's view

'I often use acupuncture because it is holistic, safely complements conventional medicine, and is successful. In 1997, 70 per cent of my patients receiving body or ear acupuncture were symptom free after an average of four treatments. It dramatically relieves acute and chronic pain, often during treatment. With chronic disease and pain, acupuncture can allow patients to reduce medication and the unpleasant side effects that accompany this. It can treat young and old, and both physical and psychological aspects of disease. I can use non-invasive techniques (laser and electrical stimulation) for those who do not want or cannot have needles. Acupressure is another alternative and patients can be taught this to control symptoms and prolong the effectiveness of treatment.'

Linda A. Tagg, Grad. Dip. Phys., MCSP, SRP, Chartered Physiotherapist and Natural Medicine Consultant

The patient's view

'I met Linda Tagg after an introduction from my GP. Having spent 14 days lying on the lounge floor, in severe spasm, with respite from the usual back treatments, my doctor asked if I would consider an alternative approach. By now, you can imagine, I was desperate.

'Linda arrived with her needles and ear studs, and, after examination, proceeded to stick her needles in all areas except where it hurt! Linda assured me that the relevant bits were being healed (perhaps by magic, thought the old sceptic, me)! Linda also suggested that the following day I would be able to move from the floor, perhaps to my feet (in your dreams, sweetheart, flashed through my mind).

'The following day, Linda arrived, stuck a few more needles in me, and then said, 'Get up.' Well, you can imagine what I was thinking. I looked out of the window. I couldn't see any stars in the sky, or shepherds, or kings – she must be mad!

'After some considerable effort on Linda's part, and some on mine, I tried to move. Slowly I moved to my knees, then to the sofa, and then to my feet. After 14 days of Valium, paramedics, chiropractors, physio … this woman with needles had achieved the impossible!

'All this was six years ago, and whenever I have any back or muscular pain now, I visit the 'Angel of Healing' for a little more acupuncture.'

Jafe Arif

The Alexander Technique

Origins

The Alexander technique was developed by Frederick Mathias Alexander who was an Australian actor working at the very beginning of the twentieth century. During the course of his acting career he developed a problem with his voice that affected his performances on stage. Intrigued as to why this was only a problem when he was on stage, and not when he was resting, he carried out some detailed self-investigation to discover the cause. Using mirrors to watch what he did when he spoke, he came to the conclusion that it was his posture that was at fault. He came to believe that the relationship between a person's head, neck and spine was the key to how the rest of the body functioned. He called it the 'primary control' and believed that when it worked in balance and harmony it had an invigorating effect on the whole person. When his own breathing and voice problems improved, he found other professional colleagues coming to him to learn the technique.

What is the Alexander technique?

The Alexander technique is more a form of education than a therapy, and consists of a combination of verbal instructions and postural guidance. The teacher instructs the pupil to adopt a much more efficient posture and to relinquish bad habits such as slumping in a chair, slouching on a sofa, sitting round-shouldered at a desk, and walking with the head bowed or slanting to one side. The Alexander technique sets out to restore in people who have chronically adopted these bad habits the ability to move with the graceful ease of a child, and to teach them how to conduct themselves with enhanced balance and poise. Teachers blame our modern working methods for many of the problems, and certainly our stressful lifestyles and sedentary occupations leave a lot to be desired.

The technique is also based on the principle that the mind and the body are inextricably linked, and that by influencing one, it is possible to have a profound effect on the other. Consequently, the tensions and strains of our everyday lives are thought to bring about poor posture and muscle tension in our bodies which then go on to cause far-reaching and nebulous symptoms generally. Furthermore, the technique maintains that by restoring postural harmony the body and mind can enjoy a spiritual and physical freedom so that even subconscious body functions, such as digestion, breathing, circulation and bowel actions, can all be improved

How does it work?

Alexander originally referred to the concept of 'primary control'. He used this term to describe the dynamic relationship between head, neck and back, which he believed was an essential indicator of a person's overall state of psychosomatic health and well-being. When tension, strain and stress occur, the natural reaction is to tense the neck muscles, pull the head back and narrow the back, a sort of primeval physical reponse designed to prepare us for a fight or flight. The Alexander technique teaches pupils to inhibit this primitive response in order to maintain perfect balance. The technique involves learning a complete discipline of postural control which can over-ride what our senses may falsely be telling us, and abolish chronic bad habits. It also involves appreciating the impact of stresses and tensions engendered by modern lifestyles and taking steps to modify these to prevent further problems.

Is the Alexander technique effective?

Pupils of the Alexander technique are generally very enthusiastic about its benefits. Having been taught its methods, they say they have been rendered free of tension, they feel lighter on their feet and they feel taller and more elegant in the way they move. Some say it has improved their co-ordination and has even enhanced their personality, making them less subservient and more self-assertive. The Alexander technique has also been used as a form of pain relief in people suffering from migraines, headaches or aching in the shoulders or arms as a result of muscle tension in the neck.

A number of medical studies have been conducted on the technique and although the studies have been small and of short duration, the results are generally encouraging and suggest that breathing problems can be improved and stress-related symptoms reduced. The technique is very popular amongst people in the performing arts, and two studies carried out on different groups of music students showed that performance stress reduction could be achieved and postural faults as well as performing abilities enhanced through regular practice of the method.

What form might the treatment take?

Teachers instruct pupils on a one-to-one basis. They will need to know what problems the pupil has been facing and how they live their lives. They will examine their posture carefully, including how they sit down in a chair and get up from a chair, how the person walks, talks, lifts and bends, and possibly even observe them as they operate a computer keyboard or play a musical instrument. The teacher then verbally guides and physically demonstrates to the pupil better ways of performing these activities. Sometimes the teacher will ask the pupil to lie flat on their back on a couch with their knees bent, and with a pad or pile of books under their head so that the neck is more or less parallel with the surface of the couch. This is the most neutral and restful position for the spine and the pupil is encouraged to be aware of how it feels. At the end of the session the pupil is given some postural exercises to conduct at home, and a plan of activity is drawn up according to the pupil's needs. The number of lessons needed will vary, but a course will often consist of 30 or so 45-minute lessons, at a frequency of 2–3 times each week.

What problems are helped by the Alexander technique?

Unlike many 'therapies', the Alexander technique does not claim to be able to remedy any specific condition or medical disorder. It does, however, claim to be able to alleviate a number of common difficulties, including chronic fatigue and tiredness, breathing disorders, musculo-skeletal aches and pains, stress-related conditions such as insomnia and palpitations, and of course problems encountered in sportsmen and women, and actors, who are held back by improper techniques or lack of maximal co-ordination.

Is it safe?

Provided the Alexander technique is taught by an experienced and qualified teacher, it is entirely safe for everybody. Healthy young children already have the natural 'primary control' which Alexander first described, but children with conditions such as muscular dystrophy, curvature of the spine, scoliosis and polio may certainly derive benefit. Pregnant women suffering from backache due to altered posture can also be taught the Alexander technique, and the elderly and the asthmatic may be helped as well.

How can I find a teacher?

It is quite possible that your NHS GP can refer you to a local teacher, but, if not, a teacher can be found by contacting the Society of Teachers of the Alexander Technique, which not only trains its members, but also involves them in a code of ethics and makes sure they are professionally indemnified and constantly updated about new developments. Members of the Society have the letters MSTAT after their names and there are some 700 or so teachers in Britain.

How much will it cost?

Each lesson costs somewhere in the region of £20–30, but it is generally recommended that a minimum of 20 lessons are booked in order to expect a meaningful result.

The sceptic's view

Of course everyone should adopt a good posture, that stands to reason, but nobody in the history of the world can ever achieve this 100 per cent of the time; nobody's chair fits them like a glove as if it were moulded to their individual spine; nobody's musculoskeletal system is developed symmetrically. Many of us may now have to sit at a desk at the office or operate a computer keyboard, but this still involves a great deal less physical stress than was involved in ploughing the land by hand two centuries ago, for example, or constructing Egyptian pyramids before the age of mechanization. Posture is important but it isn't everything. It might well be that less people would suffer from neck stiffness and respiratory problems if they walked about like African Princesses with their noses in the air and their spines ramrod straight, but unfortunately this is hardly practical. And as for those people involved in the performing arts who swear by its methods, well they're all a bit self-obsessed and narcissistic anyway, aren't they? The Alexander technique, the sceptic might conclude, is fine if you have the money and the time, but finally it is a bit of a luxury.

The therapist's view

'Teaching the Alexander technique is incredibly rewarding. It is eminently practical and can be applied to absolutely anybody in whichever situation or occupation they are in. People are amazed that they can learn so much from mere observation and analysis of how they walk, bend, sit, lift and even talk. I like to see how people perform their everyday activities both at home and at work, and by working together we can often eradicate many of the problems they find their posture and physical comportment engender. It is completely safe, especially in pregnancy when postural problems frequently cause inconvenient and uncomfortable symptoms. Although we never claim to cure any particular conditions or ailments, my clients often say that they find they have more energy, can breathe better and are more self-aware in their relationships than they ever were before discovering the Alexander technique. In particular, all kinds of joint pain emanating from the back, neck and shoulders are frequently eradicated when people are able to incorporate what they learn from the Alexander technique into their daily lives.'

Matthew Hemmings

The patient's view

'I went to the Centre for Training in North London. I was curious about the technique; all I knew was that I thought it could improve posture and lead to a general sense of well-being. My posture had suffered from too many hours spent in front of a computer screen at work – aching back and aching shoulders – and my knees had been weakened by too much strenuous activity – running several times a week, plus DIY and gardening at weekends.

'I wasn't sure what to expect. I was given a series of simple tests to check how my body moved. One of the tests involved picking up a piece of paper from the floor. I remember the first few times I picked it up my body tensed up and my knees felt sore as I crouched down. But then the practitioner told me to concentrate on my movement, not to rely on just my knees and arms to reach out for the piece of paper, but to involve the whole of my body. It took several attempts, but after a while the movement felt so graceful, so natural and, best of all, pain free! I was asked to do a series of little tests like this and, by the end of the session, not only was my posture much improved, but my body felt more relaxed. Even more important, my mind felt much calmer, too. Mentally, I felt the same as if I'd been meditating – I'd concentrated so hard on my movements that all the everyday worries in my mind had drifted away.'

Linda Powell

Aromatherapy

Origins

Aromatherapy is currently the fastest growing of all the complementary therapies, and the sale of aromatic oils is very big business, with sales running into tens of millions of pounds in recent years. The therapy is practised on a do-it-yourself basis in homes, and is prescribed in consulting rooms and administered in health and beauty salons, gymnasiums and health clinics throughout the land. These days it is even used in NHS as well as private hospitals and hospices for a whole range of symptoms, including sleep disorders, stress and anxiety, and for pain relief. In isolated cases it is even used to help women during childbirth, and patients who are suffering the unpleasant side effects of chemotherapy and radiotherapy as part of cancer treatment.

The origins of aromatherapy are as old as humankind itself, the sense of smell being one of our five basic senses, which can have far-reaching effects both consciously and unconsciously, on the individual. Smell is highly evocative of memory and can also profoundly alter our mood. It can stimulate our appetite and be a powerful pheromone with strong sexual influences and stimulatory effects. It is still fundamental to the behaviour of animals, and although it has been rather neglected by humans in the last few thousand years, it remains an important and deep-seated primeval force. Its use in therapy was described as long ago as 6,000 years, when Imhotep, the Egyptian physician, used it to help breathing and for massage purposes. Hippocrates, the Greek father of medicine, also used it in similar situations, and even used aromatic fumigations to dispel pestilence and plague.

While Europeans were almost certainly using herbs for therapeutic purposes in the Middle Ages, it was probably the Romans who first introduced aromatherapy as a method of healing, and by the eighteenth century essential oils were included in all herbalists' dispensaries and have found a place on the shelves of many physicians' consulting rooms too. The use of these essential oils diminished, however, in the nineteenth century as stronger perfumes were increasingly used, and interest focused on new developments brought about by conventional medical practitioners.

It was not until 1937 that the term 'Aromatherapy' was first coined by the French chemist Gattefossé, who used it in the title of a book which described the healing powers of essential oils. The story goes that whilst conducting an experiment in his laboratory, Gattefossé burnt his hand and plunged it into the nearest cool liquid available which happened to be a bucket of lavender oil. Noticing the speed at which the wound recovered and its freedom from infection and scarring, he investigated further and subsequently prepared all the material and groundwork for his book. During the Second World War, Dr Jean Valnet, a French army surgeon, used essential oils in the treatment of many wounded patients, and in later years,

Madame Maury took the work further, and appraised it as a holistic therapy. As such, she recommended that it should be prescribed specifically for the individual and preferably massaged into the skin as a perfect all-encompassing mind and body medicine. It was Robert Tisserand who effectively brought aromatherapy to Britain in 1969, and he started our very first training institute in the 1970s.

What is aromatherapy?

Aromatherapy literally means 'treatment using scent'. The therapy exploits the various healing capacities of essential plant oils, which may be derived from petals or other parts of the flower, from twigs of trees, and from fruit, bark, seeds or grasses. The plant oils consist of tiny droplets in the plant material which are given off in greater concentrations in particular seasons, and at certain times of the day or night. It is the evaporating oil that humans can detect through their sense of smell when it is given off as a vapour. The essential oils can be extracted from plant material by various techniques, such as solvent extraction and enfleurage, but steam distillation is by far the commonest. Using this method, over 400 different plant essences have been identified, although only about 150 are popularly used.

Each essential oil is thought to possess certain individual properties capable of producing a useful therapeutic effect in humans. All of them are antiseptic in character, and some are renowned for their anti-viral or anti-inflammatory effects while others are valued for their antidepressant, diuretic or expectorating effects. Tea tree oil, for example, has antifungal and antiseptic properties, and, as well as being a useful mouthwash, is often used to treat insect bites, grazes, candida and dandruff. Rosemary has uplifting and stimulating properties, and is often recommended to treat lassitude, general aches and pains, bad circulation and tiredness. Eucalyptus, with its anti-viral and decongestant characteristics, is employed to help with colds, coughs and chest infections.

The basic principle of aromatherapy, however, is that it is a holistic therapy and more than just the sum of its many parts. It is designed as a treatment to enhance psychological and physical health, and to promote emotional and somatic well-being. In doing so, it is thought to be helpful in avoiding any imbalance in the body's energy systems and in preventing illness and disease. The oils are usually applied by skin massage, but can also be used in inhalation therapy, in baths, or in the form of cold compresses applied directly to the skin. In addition to the overall holistic application of aromatherapy, it can be used in the clinical situation for specific ailments, although this has not been generally accepted as part of aromatherapy practice in this country, and it is used aesthetically in beauty salons for general relaxation as well as for treatment of minor skin complaints such as the generalized dry skin of ichthyosis and eczema. It is also helpful in the treatment of stretch marks, which otherwise defy treatment by any orthodox means.

How does it work?

There are many theories as to how aromatherapy might work. The most popular theory is that the sense of smell has a profound effect on a part of the brain called the limbic centre, which is also associated with powerful emotional feelings, mood and instinctive behaviour. Much has been made in recent times of neurotransmitters and hormones such as endorphins, which are the body's natural opiates and which give us a lift or a high when we are stimulated by such things as exercise or great joy. Aromatherapy is thought to stimulate the brain in similar ways, releasing neurotransmitters which have a far-reaching effect on all levels of function. Veterinary research seems to suggest that animals are susceptible to behavioural change caused by using essential oils, and it is claimed that aggressive dogs may be rendered more docile through the use of ylang-ylang and clary sage, and docile dogs rendered more aggressive exposing them to hyssop and wormwood.

The limbic system connection is all very well in theory, but why is skin massage so important? Advocates of aromatherapy tell us that the essential oils have such a fine molecular structure that they are absorbed through the skin and into the circulating bloodstream. This is unlikely, however, since the skin is specifically designed with several impervious layers expressly to keep external substances out, and we would expect, amongst all the millions of applications of aromatherapy, at least a few allergic reactions to occur if this were the case.

Is aromatherapy effective?

What little medical research has been carried out on aromatherapy appears very favourable. A French study in 1995 confirmed the idea that essential oils were antiseptic, when tea tree oil was shown to have a measurable beneficial effect in treating a particularly nasty and resistant hospital-based bacterial infection called MRSA, which inhabits the artificial ventilators that are in widespread use in Intensive Care Units and can complicate the post-operative recovery of frail, immunosuppressed patients. In the previous year, a carefully conducted, controlled trial investigated the use of aromatherapy in 100 patients who were recovering from heart surgery. Not only was the group that was treated with aromatherapy better off physiologically, but it had better overall blood pressure levels and more stable breathing and heart rate. Since some of the patients had been given massage with inactive oils to compare results, it was also claimed that the essential oils had had an active role in promoting an improved psychological effect. Interestingly, the massage on its own was shown to be useful, but the group of patients treated with nothing at all did not fare so well. Other studies on patients with intractable and recurrent epilepsy showed that it was possible to reduce the number of convulsive episodes using aromatherapy combined with post-hypnotic suggestion, and the implications of this, in terms of reducing dosages of powerful drugs with significant side effects, and the simplicity of treatment, are far reaching. Finally, an extended research project carried out by The

Central Cecil Housing Trust, which places elderly residents in sheltered accommodation, showed that aromatherapy could result in a significant reduction in anxiety, depression and pain. It helped patients with insomnia and was even shown to be of benefit to patients with the classic symptoms of senile dementia. It enabled residents to feel more peaceful and relaxed, and helped reduce their consumption of conventional analgesics and sedative drugs.

The mental health organization MIND endorses aromatherapy, amongst several complementary treatments, as an adjunct to the conventional treatment of patients with psychological problems such as depression and anxiety. Aromatherapy has even been shown to be commercially effective when used in an industrial setting: a Japanese company once used lemon fragrance, well known for its sharp and refreshing properties, to invigorate staff, while at the same time using lavender essence, known for its relaxant properties, to calm and pacify customers at the complaints desk. Not only did the staff function more efficiently, but complaints became less aggressive as well.

What form might the treatment take?

An initial consultation with an aromatherapist will usually last between one and two hours. The aroma within the consulting room is usually very noticeable to begin with, and most rooms are warm with dim or coloured lighting. There may also be some relaxing music playing. There will be a massage table, linen and towels, and obviously an array of essential oils.

Patients are asked to undress and lie on the massage table, covered by a towel for privacy. They are then asked about their medical history, their lifestyle and the kind of day they have had and its effect on their stress levels. Questions are usually asked about medication, including homeopathic remedies, as powerful essential oils are thought to be capable of neutralizing the effects of these. Based on what the therapist finds, he or she will select the right essential oils for the individual, and then blend them with a carrier oil, such as almond oil, for the purposes of the massage. Pure essential oils arc never put directly on the skin. The massage should be smooth and slow, using the traditional Swedish technique, and will generally last between 30 and 45 minutes. Some therapists will use acupressure points and incorporate some shiatsu massage (see page 300) into their technique, but generally the massage is subtle and gentle.

The therapist will avoid using certain oils if anything in the patient's history precludes them. Pregnancy, high blood pressure, a history of epilepsy or any recent operation might well be reasons for not using some oils. Treatment of patients with particularly sensitive skin should certainly be considered very carefully. In pregnancy, the toxic nature of certain essential oils, such as juniper, basil, thyme, rosemary and sage, may potentially cause damage to the unborn baby or bring about a miscarriage and therefore should not be used.

At the end of the massage, the skin should not remain greasy as most of the oil is absorbed into the superficial layers of the skin, leaving only the perfume to remind the patient of what was, hopefully, a very pleasurable form of treatment. Most patients feel relaxed and often a little emotional, and it is very common to experience some dizziness or light-headedness and lassitude after treatment. The resultant feeling is largely dependent on the essential oils used, so it is just as likely that the patient will feel invigorated if stimulating oils have deliberately been chosen.

What problems are helped by aromatherapy?

Aromatherapy is designed to work holistically, helping all aspects of a patient's emotional and physical well-being. It is especially helpful for stress-related conditions, including anxiety and depression, but is also of benefit when combined with massage for musculo-skeletal problems such as muscle aching and rheumatic pain. It is helpful for period problems, fluid retention and digestive disorders and post-natal depression, problems relating to the menopause and pre-menstrual syndrome also respond very well to it. Patients suffering from insomnia, irritability and high blood pressure will also benefit from this therapy, and even patients recovering from radiotherapy or chemotherapy as part of treatment for cancer, or those recovering from a surgical operation, may benefit. Regular aromatherapy may even enable people on long-term conventional drug therapy to reduce their dosage or come off treatment altogether, although this should only be done under the supervision and with the consent of the prescribing doctor.

Is it safe?

Aromatherapists acknowledge that essential oils are potent, and are aware that certain hazards exist. Qualified therapists will always, therefore, use the oils with caution especially in situations such as pregnancy, high blood pressure, epilepsy, diabetes and skin conditions. Therapists should also be aware that some oils may interact with certain homeopathic medicines, and that others can be photo-sensitizing, causing skin damage when the patient is subsequently exposed to sunlight. The citrus oils, orange, lemon and bergamot fall into this category, for example. Other oils, like cinnamon bar, are more likely to cause allergic skin reactions than others. The oils should always be kept out of the reach of young children, too, as swallowing them could prove fatal. Anyone indulging in do-it-yourself therapy should be aware of the potency of certain essential oils; just because they are on unrestricted sale in Britain, and often carry no danger warnings, does not mean they may be used with impunity.

How can I find an aromatherapist?

Aromatherapy oils can be bought over the counter in high-street shops, supermarkets and chemists, and are therefore widely available. Some so-called aromatherapy oils are entirely synthetic and will not possess the same qualities as the pure products. The Aromatherapy Trade Council (ATC) was established in 1993, and is a self-regulating organization representing three-quarters of all suppliers of essential oils. It has defined an essential oil as 'an aromatic volatile substance extracted by distillation'; an absolute oil as 'obtained by solvent extraction'; and an aromatherapy oil as 'the essential oil mixed with a carrier oil'. However, it has not yet defined what an aromatherapy *product* is, so consumers and trading standards officers are likely to remain bemused. Some aromatherapy products will contain hardly any essential oil whatsoever, merely a synthetic fragrance designed to appeal to the customer's sense of smell. Price varies enormously even amongst the pure essential oils. Since it takes about 100 kg (220 lb) of lavender to produce 3 kg (6½ lb) of oil, lavender oil remains reasonably inexpensive. But it apparently takes 8 million jasmine flowers, selected at dawn, to produce a mere 1 kg (2¼ lb) of jasmine oil, so jasmine oil in its purest form is very expensive.

Therapists themselves may or may not be qualified. At present the therapy is unregulated, and anyone can claim to be an expert. The Aromatherapy Organizations Council (AOC) represent a total of 26,000 therapists who probably constitute nine-tenths of the practitioners in this country. However, there are many different types of registration, some therapists having undertaken courses lasting only a few hours, while others have studied for up to two years. Any potential patient who wishes to proceed cautiously would be advised to select a therapist trained at an AOC approved college of aromatherapy, although many consumers are content to receive treatment from someone who clearly has not had expert training for any significant length of time, but whose manner, enthusiasm and ability make up for that.

How much will it cost?

For one and a half hours of aromatherapy massage, most people would expect to pay somewhere in the region of £40. Many people, whose long-standing complaints are alleviated by the treatment, choose regular follow-up sessions and are usually offered a special rate to suit their purse.

The sceptic's view

Nice pong, great massage, not so convinced about the therapeutic properties though! Conventional doctors have been using eucalyptus in inhalant products since time immemorial, but to extend claims of the therapeutic value of essential oils into the realms of heart disease and cancer is far-fetched. Thousands of people have jumped on the bandwagon of this admittedly pleasant therapy, but this just goes to show that anybody can practise it because just as there is no powerful benefit, there is no powerful risk either. If the essential oil really did penetrate the skin as it is claimed to do, hundreds of people would by now have suffered nasty and all-encompassing allergies, and secondary toxic reactions would be two-a-penny. Surely, too, with therapists spending several hours a day applying different essential oils to different clients, they must be thoroughly confusing their own bodies by their effects! Can a therapist apply relaxing lavender and rosemary at 12 midday, and stimulating lemon and eucalyptus at 1.30 p.m. , and yet remain totally unaffected? Or do the holistic aromatherapists merely explain this away by saying that the oils have not been selected for themselves as an individual? Therapists also tell us their products are very potent, yet where are the patient information leaflets which conventional drugs have to carry with them when they are prescribed, and why isn't the treatment properly regulated as this would seem to suggest is required? One particular idea perpetrated by aromatherapists will certainly make the sceptic laugh. It is that some oils such as lavender and lemon, are 'adaptogenic' implying that they can adapt to whatever it is the human body demands of them in any given situation. How clever, the disbeliever might think: a truly magic formula uniquely dispensed by sorcerers for the delectation of believers in the supernatural.

The therapist's view

'Aromatherapy is my favourite therapy because I love working with the oils. They leave me feeling calmer, happier and uplifted physically and

emotionally. Many a time I have floated out of my treatment room as high as a kite, depending on which euphoric oils I have been using. i. e. ylang-ylang and clary sage.

'The essential oils can be utilized in many way, including massage techniques, perfumes, aromatic baths, skincare preparations, compresses, masks, inhalations and douches. Certain oils can also be used on infants and children.

'All oils and treatments should be chosen with care, ensuring that any medical condition is known and treatments are carried out with the co-operation of the client's medical practitioner.

'Essential oils have a powerful life-force and must be diluted and used under the supervision of a qualified aromatherapist.'

Phillippa Stacy, MIFA, ISPA
Tutor and Therapist

The patient's view

'I am a wife, a mum, a grandmother and a businesswoman – I also have psoriasis. My life is busy, to say the least, but that's the way I like it. To keep my energy levels up I follow a low-fat diet, walk my dogs for exercise and once a month have an aromatherapy massage which I find totally relaxing and enjoyable. This is time spent for me and the benefits have a positive effect on my state of mind and body. I find that my psoriasis is stress-related – not necessarily related to worry but to the stresses of everyday life. Any kind of relaxation promotes a calmness within me which keeps my psoriasis comfortable and controlled. My therapist understands this, and we work together to achieve the best results for me.'

J. Hallum

Art Psychotherapy (including Music Therapy and Drama Therapy)

Origins

Most artistic pursuits represent types of self-expression, and are therefore useful in helping to rehabilitate the mentally ill and treat those with psychological and emotional disorders. Music, dancing and drawing are wonderful emotional outlets, the benefits of which became apparent during the Second World War, when they were helpful in rehabilitating wounded soldiers. Such activities provided an opportunity of setting up the relationship with medical and nursing staff which enabled healing to follow. Over the years, different art therapies have been accepted by the NHS, and recognized post-graduate training in art therapy became established in the 1970s. Finally, in 1982, the Diploma in Art Therapy was formally recognized by the Department of Health, something for which the British Association of Art Therapists had campaigned hard.

What is art psychotherapy?

Art psychotherapy uses a number of different psychotherapies to encourage people to express themselves and to overcome psychological problems. It promotes tentative discussions about how people feel about themselves and, of course, about how others within their environment react to them. Broadly speaking, art psychotherapy is designed to grant people control over their own lives, by enabling them to express in a different way things that they have never been able to put across before. By doing this in a safe and unthreatening situation, they are often able to overcome emotional and physical disabilities, thus promoting their independence and personal growth. The particular therapy a patient uses is generally not critical, although a skilled therapist may feel that one type will enable an individual patient to express their emotions more effectively than another.

How does it work?

Art therapy encourages patients to express themselves through drawing, painting, pottery, sculpture and a variety of other art forms. The therapist delves into the significance of what has been created so that an insight into 'where the patient is coming from' can be gleaned. This is a good way of establishing a discussion with patients who find it difficult to make close and lasting relationships. The art work created is confidential and any hidden feelings connected with the work are only ever treated sensitively and sympathetically.

Drama therapy involves groups of people in role play, enabling them to act out imaginary scenes with which they can identify, as a means of furthering their education, creativity and personal growth. Social interaction can be practised both in a real or metaphorical way, and attitudes, principles and emotions can be teased out and developed.

Music therapy is now not only carried out in hospitals, but in special and residential schools as well, since everyone can appreciate and be moved by music, however badly physically or mentally handicapped they are. Some patients actually communicate through a musical language peculiar to them, and music therapy itself is central to the work of many occupational therapists, speech therapists and physiotherapists. This form of treatment is medically orientated, with the same goals and objectives as other art therapies and can be beneficial to people who have suffered strokes and have dysphasia (difficulty with speech). It can also be helpful in calming hyperactive children and patients with dementia.

Dance movement therapy uses physical movement to promote the expression of emotions, and as such is often applicable to people with anxiety and depression, as well as people who are severely disturbed or even psychotic. Children with learning difficulties, AIDS sufferers, and those with eating disorders, have benefited from dance movement therapy, and the work is carried out in special schools, residential homes, day centres and hospitals.

Is art psychotherapy effective?

Art psychotherapy is acknowledged by many conventional doctors working in NHS hospitals as being highly beneficial to certain groups of patients, and scientific research appears to endorse this. Well-documented clinical studies have shown that art psychotherapy can effectively reduce anxiety in a number of medical settings, and can even influence blood pressure and pulse rates in patients recovering from coronary bypass surgery.

What form might the treatment take?

The type of treatment given can be varied and diverse. It can be practised on a one-to-one basis with the therapist or occur in groups, and may be carried out in a number of different clinical locations. Therapy generally continues for several months and hospital in-patients with chronic disorders may enjoy the benefits of art psychotherapy for several years if it is considered appropriate.

What problems are helped by art psychotherapy?

Although many types of emotional and psychological disorder can benefit from art psychotherapy, its effects are most rewarding in people whose fears and anxieties hold them back from maximizing their full potential, perhaps because they are handicapped by intensely negative thoughts or low self-esteem. It is also of benefit to people who find it difficult to form close, meaningful relationships, and it helps those with learning disorders, and even people suffering from dementia or organic psychiatric disease. Any patient without normal speech can learn new channels of communication through this therapy, and children, especially, thrive on the non-threatening and fun side of it.

Is it safe?

Certainly all these therapies are safe; the important thing is that they are appropriate and tailored to the individual patient.

How can I find an art psychotherapist?

Although it is not a generally known fact, art therapy has been practised by qualified, skilled individuals belonging to reputable professional bodies for many years. The Department of Health recognizes these therapies, and the qualifications which go with them. The initials RATh stand for Registered Art Therapist, RMTh for Registered Music Therapist and SRMTh for State Registered Music Therapist. Music therapists are not only qualified musicians, but have also had a long training in clinical care; other therapists working in the fields of dance, art and drama have not only graduated in their specialist subjects, but may have qualifications in additional subjects such as sociology or psychology. Your NHS doctor can refer you to any type of art therapist, or the relevant individual associations can be approached for a list of qualified therapists in your area.

How much will it cost?

Hopefully these therapies can be obtained on the NHS. Private art psychotherapy usually costs in the region of £20–30 an hour and some therapists run weekend courses for £100–150.

The sceptic's view

The total disbeliever would probably recommend to patients that they listen to a CD of their favourite music rather than referring them to some airy-fairy art therapist who would plonk away at the piano or splash oil paints abstractly on to a canvas, but then many a medical sceptic has never set foot in an art therapy session, and would in any case have little contact with patients suffering from learning disabilities, mental illness or chronic physical disease. However, the sceptic would probably acknowledge that art therapy is a field about which he knows very little, and that it is a particularly difficult type of work into which even the best and most advanced modern medical technology cannot effectively penetrate. The sceptic might also take the view that since not very much else can be done for these types of patients they might just as well be kept occupied and stimulated by the art therapists rather than sitting around the hospital wards getting in the nursing staff's way.

The therapist's view

'As a music therapist, I have been deeply influenced by both the various client groups with which I have worked and also by the institutions within which I have worked. Initially in my career I worked for the NHS with children, adolescents and adults with mental health problems. Over the past six years or so I have worked with those who are living with, or who are affected by, terminal illness – mainly HIV/AIDS, but also with various forms of cancer.

'With most clients, the main tool of my work is creative musical improvization, using a wide range of tuned and untuned percussion instruments I encourage the client to make music with me. It's not that I feel able to learn how the client may be feeling by how they play music, rather that through a process of intense listening and acceptance, we can both begin to be able to experience ourselves in music. So rather than "What is this music about for this person?", I find myself asking "How is this person benefiting from experiencing themselves as being musical?" The core of this way of working is the realization that no matter what may happen to us in life, whatever problems befall us, our responses to music always remain healthy.

'There are two common responses from people with regard to working in this way. The first is that people surprise themselves – by the quality of what they create. The second is that people comment on having a new experience of themselves. When working with those who are dying, these can be significant experiences; as one patient who was close to death put it: "When we're improvising music, I've never felt so alive!"'

Nigel Alan Hartley MA, BMus(Hons), Dip N-RMTh
Senior Music Therapist

The patient's view

'Music therapy helped to break down the barriers after my diagnosis as HIV positive. It offered me the chance, and the challenge, to set out on a previously unattempted journey of creative self-exploration at the moment when I could have retreated into passivity and despair. Music is so big, it always has room, and a vocabulary, for whatever one wants to express. Yet the silence it incorporates, and out of which it grows, is acutely charged with the potential for listening and being heard. During the sessions I never felt my personality, or my situation, being diminished by the imposition of a simplistic methodology. Sometimes I had to overcome the fear of making a self-exposing gesture, but was always rewarded with the grace of meaningful response. By means of this journey, with the music therapist as a constant support and companion. I became the creator, but also the sharer, of beauty.'

A. Robbins

Autogenic Training

Origins

Autogenic training, or AT, was devised by Dr Johannes Schultz, a German psychiatrist and neurologist working in Berlin in the 1920s. He was interested in the fact that people under hypnosis became deeply relaxed and could escape the various psychosomatic ailments which disrupted their lives. He was also very much aware of the physical changes which people exhibited under hypnosis: most subjects feel warm and heavy in this heightened state of self-awareness and are able to switch off that part of the nervous system, the sympathetic nervous system, which becomes so active when stimulated by the strains and stresses of today's crazy world. By allowing its equal and opposite counterpart, the parasympathetic nervous system, to come more into play, these physical changes can be produced. AT was introduced in Britain in the 1970s and is still practised as an effective self-taught stress-relieving method.

What is autogenic training?

Autogenic training involves deep relaxation brought about by concentrating the mind on ways of reversing the consequences of stress and strain, both physically and psychologically. It is similar to meditation as well as self-hypnosis; in fact the word 'autogenic' literally means 'self-induced'. Unlike self-hypnosis, however, where suggestions are introduced to the subconscious mind, in AT the mind concentrates on thoughts or feelings which promote deep relaxation. A repertoire of straightforward exercises is employed to turn off the physiological stress response, and a large number of biological changes, which have been measured qualitatively, take place in the body during these exercises.

How does it work?

Essentially, AT works by influencing the autonomic (unconscious) nervous system through higher mental functions. Just as a fright or a shock produces an increase in the pulse rate and palpitations, sweaty palms and rapid breathing, so calming the mind can reduce the respiration and pulse rate and change the activity of the glands and hormonal system. Many of today's common stress-related ailments, such as insomnia, nausea, under- or over-eating and tremor or panic attacks, are the result of living in today's frenetic rat race, and can be alleviated when the parasympathetic nervous system is allowed to function properly. The problem is that in everyday life it is only the sympathetic nervous system which is constantly stimulated, the parasympathetic system only having a significant effect on our bodies when we are totally at rest, which is rare. AT balances these two system, which are supposed to be equal and opposite so that the body can self-heal. The techniques 'of autogenic training involve the use of two lots of exercises. The first relaxes the patient by introducing a type of self-hypnosis, and the second, called 'intentional exercises' are designed to release physical and psychological tension. These may involve practices as diverse as screaming, crying, hitting cushions or even shadow-boxing.

Is autogenic training effective?

It is widely accepted that autogenic training may be very useful in alleviating any symptoms which are stress-related. Used for insomnia, tension headaches, palpitations and irritable bowel syndrome, AT has also been shown to be of benefit for high blood pressure. A five-year study completed in 1988 showed that in mild hypertension, patients did better with AT than they did using a placebo, needed less medication and took less overall sick leave. In another study in 1994, patients suffering from panic attacks and anxiety also reported less symptoms after AT, and the benefits were still significant three months later.

What form might the treatment take?

AT can be given either on a one-to-one basis or in small groups. As in any orthodox consultation, the patient provides information about his or her complaint and medical history, and the therapist enquires about general lifestyle and the administration of any medication. The exercises are then taught on a once-a-week basis for, say, two months, each session lasting about one hour. The patient is encouraged to practise the techniques at home, and patients are also warned about simple 'autogenic discharges', which are a temporary exacerbation of current or previous problems, and which are generally regarded as a kind of exorcism of pre-existing factors.

What problems are helped by AT?

This technique does not specifically aim to remedy particular diseases, but is designed to help the well-being of each patient holistically. It is, however, probably best at treating stress-related conditions, including colitis, irritable bowel syndrome, asthma, high blood pressure, anxiety and panic disorders, insomnia, palpitations, premenstrual syndrome, bladder problems, infertility, tension headache, migraine and even epilepsy and drug addiction.

Is it safe?

AT is entirely safe in the hands of a qualified teacher. Patients not considered suitable for treatment are those with personality disorders and organic psychoses, such as schizophrenia.

How can I find an AT teacher?

A list of qualified teachers may be obtained from the British Association for Autogenic Training and Therapy (BAFATT). Autogenic training teachers are usually trained in psychotherapy and may well have undergone further training for up to two years.

How much will it cost?

Depending on whether you are taught individually or in a group, the cost of a course of 10 or so AT lessons will be between £200 and £300. The charge will depend on where you live, but if it is something you desperately want to try but cannot afford, ask your own family doctor about a possible referral to the Royal London Homeopathic Hospital, where some training takes place for this purpose. BAFATT ensures that therapists adopt a recognized code of ethics, and that teachers are subject to disciplinary procedures. As individual practitioners, AT therapists are covered by professional indemnity insurance.

The sceptic's view

Since stress is a normal physiological response to any kind of challenge, and is not necessarily harmful, the typical sceptic is likely to ask whether autogenic training is necessary at all. Obviously some people are more tense and more prone to stress-related symptoms than others, and those people who are the most conscientious, the born worriers of this world, do seem to have trouble winding down. But there is nothing a brisk walk over the moors, a vigorous game of squash or a mad night's dancing should not put right. In fact, the true sceptic would say that physical exercise is a much better antidote to an over-dominant sympathetic nervous system, than lying completely still and getting your mind to relax your body the hard way.

Autogenic training may reduce blood pressure slightly, but it will not reduce it enough in moderate or severe cases to enable an 'at-risk' patient to avoid medication. Who are the seriously stressed out members of our society who can afford ten one-hour sessions plus 15 minutes three times a day, to practise the techniques out of their busy schedule? It is a nice idea to *think* your hands warm on a cold day and motivate your mind to make your bowels work more frequently, but the sceptic might view the real benefit of AT as serving to keep the anxiety-prone phobic clear of the overworked GP's surgery.

The therapist's view

'I have been using autogenic training (AT) both for individuals and for groups in a corporate setting for many years with highly satisfying results. On an individual basis, AT has helped people with anxiety and even chronic forms of depression, and anyone with stress-related symptoms, such as irritable bowel syndrome, tension headache, high blood pressure, insomnia, pre-menstrual syndrome and asthma, have all benefited. Even predominantly physical symptoms, such as bladder complaints, epilepsy, colitis, infertility and rheumatism, have improved in patients I have instructed because there is clearly an involuntary component produced by an over-active nervous system. In a corporate setting, personnel departments have noticed a reduction in sick leave taken by staff, and the employees themselves are delighted that the companies have taken the trouble at their own expense to make this beneficial form of therapy available to them in their lunch-breaks. I will continue my work with AT exercises because I find it extremely rewarding and effective.'

B. Hennessy

The patient's view

'I had put up with irritable bowel syndrome (IBS) on and off for several years and was sick and tired of my job, which was immensely stressful and made me irritable, tense and aggressive. I wasn't sleeping well, my pre-menstrual syndrome was worse, and because of the IBS my whole life seemed to revolve around the loo and my bad temper. I started using autogenic exercises, which soon helped me to appreciate the physiological changes which happened in my body when I learnt how to relax properly. I quickly became aware of unconscious things, like my heart-beat, my breathing and even my insides. Autogenic training also helped me to release physical and emotional tension by giving me permission, as it were, in a group of like-minded people to shout, scream and cry. The best thing of all was punching and throwing pillows which on one occasion left us all falling about laughing. Now my IBS is well under control, and I am a much nicer person to be with and work with.'

Mary Dollan

Ayurvedic Medicine

Origins

The word 'ayurveda' comes from two Sanskrit words meaning 'the science of life'. Some 5,000 years ago, this sophisticated system of health care was developed by the wise men of ancient India, and their combination of science and philosophy covered many of the modern components of sickness and health. One of the first texts, originating in about 2500 BC, the *Charaka Samhita*, described how the body was made up of cells, and how disease could be spread by micro-organisms. Another document, the *Susrutha Samhita*, talked about surgical techniques and equipment, and its coverage of the subject of hygiene pre-dated that vital breakthrough of aseptic technique in surgery, which made such a huge difference to the survival of patients in the middle of the nineteenth century. It was way ahead of its time even then, but ayurvedic medicine remains the traditional system of medicine practised by many doctors in India and Sri Lanka. Ayurvedic medicine is widespread in all of Asia and in Asian communities; most of the ayurvedic practitioners in Britain work in areas such as London, Birmingham, Bradford and Leicester for this reason, and this is where the popularity of ayurvedic medicine has spread from since it was first introduced to this country in the mid-1970s.

What is ayurvedic medicine?

The complex holistic system of health care called ayurveda deals with the physical, mental, spiritual and emotional aspect of health and disease. Like traditional Chinese medicine, it does more than try to prevent and correct disease – it encourages us to fulfil our true potential and to lead a meaningful and balanced life. Essentially, the ayurvedic principle is that we are all one with the universe, and that we consist of part of the life-force or 'prana' of the universe. On one level our bodies are simply physical shells, but on another we are tiny parts of a universe consisting of billions of individual organisms of vibrating energy.

Ayurvedic practitioners recognize that treatment must be tailored to suit the individual patient as there is no universal prescription for well-being that suits everybody. The 'prana' controls every process within our bodies, and the practitioner's acumen is based upon his ability to discover each patient's constitution and to locate the exact source of their energy imbalance, so that the correct solution can be found.

How does it work?

Ayurveda has been developed to promote good health and well-being through a combination of herbal medicine, meditation, yoga, astrology and dietary advice. It has components of many different complementary therapies, including relaxation, spiritual and physical exercise, aromatherapy and herbalism, and in many ways it is similar to traditional Chinese medicine, but the life-force in ayurveda is known as 'ojas', the equivalent of the Chinese chi. Instead of trying to treat illness once it has been established, ayurveda is designed to prevent disease by strengthening the individual's constitution and the way it relates to his or her energy balance. Each of us balances three vital energies in the body, termed the three 'doshas' – 'vatha', 'pitha' and 'kaptha'. Individual patients are controlled by one or more dominant doshas, so that they might be a kaptha type, a vatha type or a pitha type, or they might be a combination type, such as vatha–pitha or kaptha–vatha, and so on. The belief is that the doshas impinge on every facet of everyday life, and can alter personality and can affect outlook as well as physical constitution. For example, the doshas can affect the colour of your skin, your size and shape, and how you react to certain elements in your diet.

The three doshas work best in harmony, as each has its unique role in the body. Pitha relates to fire and water, and is generally in control of metabolism, being responsible for the digestive juices in the body, the enzymes, stomach acid and bile. Kaptha is related to earth and water, and controls secretions from the mucous membranes, the phlegm, lymphatic flow, fluids and fatty tissues. Vatha relates to the body's energy and is the driving force that stimulates the nervous system and controls the speed at which various body functions are carried out. The three doshas are kept in balance by our nutritional intake, the amount of exercise we take, the elimination of unhealthy waste substances, and a stable emotional and spiritual health. In ayurvedic philosophy every individual is born in the 'prakruthi' state and, at that moment, the doshas are perfectly balanced. As we go through life, however, the influence of the external environment, our diet, stress, and emotional and physical damage alter this perfect state by unbalancing the doshas, and the individual then reaches the 'vikruthi' state, when equilibrium is lost and ill-health and illness result. Practitioners of ayurvedic medicine attempt to bring patients back to the prakruthi state. They do this by adjusting diet, altering lifestyle, and by detoxification.

Practitioners also talk about the five elements – fire, water, air, earth and ether (or space). These five elements are present in everything, including ourselves, where they control every part and function of the body as well as the senses. The elements are governed by the energy of fire or 'agni', which, when functioning normally, maintains every bodily function. Imbalances in the doshas, dietary or sexual excess, and emotional turmoil can all unbalance 'agni', resulting in ill-health. For example, fluid retention brought about by excessive drinking would mean that too much kaptha has a negative effect on 'agni', resulting in a sluggish digestive process causing indigestion and heaviness. On the other hand, too much of the vatha dosha can lead to cramps, flatulence and altered bowel habit. 'Agni' also controls the efficient functioning of the three 'malas' which are the body's three excretory systems of urine, faeces and sweat.

Another interesting part of ayurvedic philosophy is that emotional repression can lead to illnesses such as irritable bowel syndrome or food allergies, through the production and build-up of toxins in the body. Apprehension and anxiety are associated with vatha, which alters efficient regular contractions within the large intestine, leading to abdominal cramps and bloating. Loss of absorptive powers, and a build-up of toxins, can lead to food allergies and cause food cravings likely to bring about further physical imbalance. According to ayurvedic teachers, where physical health is often treated with dietary and lifestyle alteration, emotional difficulties may often respond better to meditation and yoga.

Is ayurvedic medicine effective?

While no scientific controlled studies have been conducted in the West to prove the efficacy of ayurvedic medicine, limited studies performed overseas have pointed to its usefulness in the area of controlling hyperglycaemia (excess blood sugar in those with diabetes) and in helping patients with Parkinson's disease using an ayurvedic seed powder called Mucuna. Dr Deepak Chopra, who trained as a consultant endocrinologist in the United States, has published many books on ayurvedic medicine, and his ability to combine Western and ancient Indian medicine has attracted widespread popularity and respect both at home and abroad.

What form might the treatment take?

As in conventional medicine, the consultation with the ayurvedic practitioner consists of diagnosis and treatment. To reach the initial diagnosis, the patient's medical history is taken, and details are elicited about the patient's symptoms, outlook, lifestyle and social habits. The patient's previous medical history, and that of his or her parents is also usually discussed. The practitioner will also want to know what the patient was like as a child and as a teenager in order to determine the patient's prakruthi state, so that he or she can then identify the dominant dosha. The patient will be asked about their career, their family, their preferences and dislikes, their level of physical activity and their diet, and then specific questions relating to digestion, nervous system and appetite may be asked.

The physical part of the examination may take about half an hour, beginning with observation of the patient's demeanour, behaviour, and also taking into account colour, complexion, build and speech. In particular, the tongue, eyes, lips and nails will be examined for signs of any doshic imbalance. Someone who is very talkative, for example, would be classified as a vatha person, whereas someone who had a heavy coating on their tongue might be considered to be under the influence of the kaptha dosha. The pulse diagnosis, which is called the 'nadi shastra', is then taken with the practitioner's three little fingers feeling for three pulse points at each of the patient's wrists. It is said that a good ayurvedic practitioner can detect up to 30 different pulse qualities in this manner.

Once a diagnosis has been reached, a treatment can be selected. The first type equates to detoxification of the body, as this is a fundamental facet of ayurvedic medicine and is used before any remedial treatment is contemplated. The detoxification is designed to correct any imbalance of the doshas, to restore proper function of the digestive system, and to eradicate any environmental poisons from the body. The two-day detoxification treatment consists of herbal oils being massaged into the skin over 'marma' points that equate to acupressure points in Chinese medicine, and steam baths, to promote the eradication of toxins through the sweat glands. A more intricate form of detoxification is called 'panchakarma', which may involve oil enema therapy, herbal laxative or enema treatment, inhalation therapy and, in some cases, even therapeutic vomiting.

Once the detoxification treatment has been completed, the patient is often prescribed mineral or herbal treatments to correct any doshic imbalance. 'Samana' treatment uses products derived from herbs or plants, from bark, seeds, fruits, leaves and roots. Other substances used in ayurvedic medicine include animal products, minerals and sea shells. They may come in the form of a liquid or as dried herbs, but they can also be provided in powder or tablet form. Ingredients are chosen according to the desired effect they will have in correcting imbalances in the doshas. A typical prescription would be made up of a number of different herbs to which water is added and the liquid then boiled until it becomes much more concentrated. Typically, the medication would then be taken two or three times a day. Individual ingredients would be chosen for their remedial effect on any dominant dosha. For example, spices whose taste is bitter, such as turmeric and hot spices, such as cayenne and cinnamon would be chosen for patients who needed to reduce kaptha and who might be suffering from sinusitis, bronchitis or catarrh. The patient might also be encouraged to restrict their intake of cold drinks, which would have the opposite effect and increase kaptha.

In addition to detoxification and samana treatment, meditation, dietary advice and yoga might also be recommended according to the patient's needs. Further appointments would be suggested, depending on the particular problem that is being treated, and might typically occur once a fortnight or once a month.

What problems are helped by ayurvedic medicine?

Since ayurvedic medicine is a holistic form of treatment, almost everything falls under its therapeutic umbrella. Designed to create well-being and stimulate maximum health, it is particularly recommended for chronic fatigue, joint problems and headaches, and for skin conditions such as eczema, psoriasis and acne. Heartburn, stomach ulcers and irritable bowel syndrome are also often treated by ayurveda as are menopausal symptoms, period complaints, pre-menstrual syndrome and sexual difficulties, including infertility. Constipation, water retention and even circulatory disorders can be improved with ayurvedic medicine.

Is it safe?

Some traditional herbal products may potentially be contaminated with toxic substances like heavy metal particles, and the rigorous detoxification of panchakarma would certainly not be suitable for pregnant women, the very elderly, or people prone to fainting. Herbs, too, even when not adulterated with extraneous pollutants, can have far-reaching medical effects, and so anything taken by mouth should always be correctly prescribed and taken in the appropriate amount and form. Any reputable ayurvedic practitioner would also not encourage the patient to abandon any orthodox therapy they might be taking.

How can find an ayurvedic practitioner?

The Ayurvedic Medical Association UK keeps a list of qualified practitioners, of which there are just a handful at the current time. They have all undergone six years of training at universities in either India or Sri Lanka and most of them work in Britain in regions where there are substantial Asian communities. There are many other ayurvedic practitioners, however, who have taken crash courses in ayurveda and who may not be registered with the association. Other centres have been set up by the Maharishi Mahesh Yogi, who also set up the transcendental meditation movement, from where Maharishi Ayur-Veda is practised. All practitioners who are registered with the Ayurvedic Medical Association UK have to abide by the Association's code of conduct, and carry a form of professional indemnity.

How much will it cost?

The cost of the initial consultation, lasting at least one hour, will be somewhere around £50, and subsequent treatments are usually charged at about £30 per session. Maharishi Ayur-Veda may be more expensive than this. Full detoxification, lasting up to three days, may cost up to £400, with herbal remedy prices on top, averaging about £10 a month.

The sceptic's view

The sceptic might argue that ayurvedic medicine is still the most commonly used traditional form of medicine in parts of India and Sri Lanka simply because it is extremely cheap, and for most there is no alternative. The highly imaginative concept that your constitution and personality are decided by how your mother and father are feeling when you are conceived is interesting, but nobody has come up with any real evidence to prove that this is the case. A fanciful philosophy based on mysticism, and with no scientific evidence that it works, ayurvedic medicine clearly should not be used for people with serious illness, like cancer, or for those who need surgery, although it should not do very much harm to people for whom conventional therapy has little to offer. The disbeliever will probably have little interest in the notion of detoxification, despite this having become incredibly fashionable amongst people of celebrity status, and they would almost certainly raise an eyebrow at the considerable expense of herbal and oil enemas and therapeutic vomiting.

The therapist's view

The growing popularity of ayurvedic medicine speaks for itself. Patients who have been failed by orthodox medicine with recurrent and inconvenient symptoms such as irritable bowel syndrome, ME (myalgic encephalomyelitis), migraine and skin-related conditions, can obtain great benefit, but also need considerable time and assessment to have the underlying causes of their difficulties properly explored. The whole philosophy is a soothing and interesting one, a completely different way of thinking about oneself, one's health and freedom from disease. Detoxification in our modem world, surrounded as we are by environmental poisons and pollutants, is a form of treatment which makes people feel cleansed and treated from within, and the remedies are generally gentle and natural. Ayurvedic medicine also is a form of treatment practised largely by doctors trained in orthodox ways and it therefore lends itself well to conditions which even the most academic specialist doctors sometimes fail to remedy.

The patient's view

'I have hepatitis C with progressive liver disease and related chronic fatigue. It is believed that I contracted it through a blood transfusion received in a hospital in America some years ago. Shortly after its diagnosis I was treated with the best available Western medication – injections of Interferon Alfa 2b. The Interferon treatment failed to kill the hepatitis C virus, and the side effects were severe, including extreme fatigue and depression.

'I became unable to perform my professional duties. My ability level to carry on normal living was reduced to approximately 25 per cent. Jogging, skiing, hiking, bicycling, international travelling and socializing, which were my life, were no longer possible. Whereas I had previously jogged 2–3 miles a day, I was now confined to very short 5–10-minute walks. My immune system was compromised to the point where I incurred frequent and severe cases of flu and bad colds which lasted for long periods and required bed rest.

'I have also been afflicted with a benign enlarged prostate and related bladder irregularities. These conditions produced frequent high pain levels for which large dosages of Western pain medication were prescribed. The side effects of these prescriptions resulted in stomach and intestinal disorders.

'In looking for alternative solutions to my problems I undertook a programme of acupuncture, herbal medicine and ayurveda medicine under the direction of Dr Godagama in London, England.

'I am now very pleased to report my fatigue levels have been reduced significantly to the point where I am able to resume approximately 60–70 per cent of my professional and personal activities. Frequency of flu and colds has been reduced to near-normal levels and elevated liver enzymes have been reduced to low or tolerable.

'After 3–4 years of near immobility, I am now looking forward to continued improvement and resumption to previously normal levels of my life's activities, with continual treatment consisting of detoxification programmes, herbal medicinal prescriptions and correct diet.'

Edward Gartland

Bach Flower Remedies

Origins

Dr Edward Bach (pronounced 'batch') was a physician and bacteriologist and later a homeopath, who ran a thriving practice in Harley Street until 1930 when he gave it all up at the age of 43 to pursue his growing interest in flower remedies. He had always been more interested in people than their illnesses, and he had come to believe that personality and character had an overwhelming influence over general health. For years, Dr Bach had escaped the confines of London to go for long walks in the countryside and was struck by how walking through woods and fields in the fresh air could relax and revitalize him. He was drawn to particular flowers especially and began to experiment with the effects of dew taken from the flowers he came across. Starting with an initial 12 remedies, he added more by soaking flower petals in spring water, and eventually developed 38 flower remedies for the benefit of every possible personality, state of mind and emotional state.

Other flower remedies exist, but the ones made famous by Dr

Bach are very successfully produced to this day by The Edward Bach Centre in Oxfordshire, at the house where the founder once lived. The 38 Bach Flower Remedies were initially regarded as a complete health system, and Bach himself insisted before his death that in the interests of keeping the system simple, no further remedies should be added. He had also categorized patients' emotional difficulties into seven basic groups, namely fear, apathy, loneliness, oversensitivity, despair, too much concern for other people, uncertainty and indecision.

What are Bach flower remedies?

Bach flower remedies comprise 38 small bottles of tincture that are widely available. The remedies are capable of lifting a patient's mood thus enabling them to improve their health, cure any negative thoughts and promote healing. The remedies are supposed to work on a vibrational level within the body, just as in homeopathy (see page 202), and by abolishing anxiety, tension, stress, grief and frustration can make people better by removing those factors which bring about illness in the first place.

The remedies are produced by one of two methods, the sun method and the boiling method. In the former, flower petals are put in a bowl of spring water and left in strong sunlight for several hours. Later, the energized water is transferred into small bottles half filled with brandy, a practice which is designed to permanently preserve the flower essence. This is then regarded as the Mother Tincture and can later be diluted, again with brandy, to make the commercially available remedies, which are sold in distinctive little brown bottles. The boiling method is used for remedies requiring a more powerful extraction process. Parts of the flowering plant are boiled for half an hour in spring water, and again the liquid essence is mixed with brandy before being bottled.

How do the remedies work?

Like homeopathic medicines, Bach flower remedies contain no

detectable or recognizable ingredients from the original plant or flower. Flower therapists explain that each remedy contains merely the imprint of the flower from which it was derived, and that the energy contained within the remedy acts as a catalyst to trigger the body's innate healing powers.

Some of the essences are known as 'type remedies', and are specially selected to suit the individual patient's particular characteristics and personality. Type remedies are taken when any negative thoughts or emotions are threatening to damage the patient's health. Many of the remedies have a very specific application, whereas others can be used for a number of different emotions. Vine, for example, might be used by strong, dominant and ambitious people who are natural leaders, but who may be at risk of becoming quite obsessive and dictatorial. The vine remedy is supposed to enable them to be more aware of other people's feelings, and to make them more empathetic without detracting from their positive qualities of leadership. Honeysuckle is used for people who are too backward-looking and unwilling to accept new developments. Impatiens is a remedy which helps impatient, intolerant people adopt a more relaxed and more laid-back approach to life. Rescue remedy is possibly the most commonly used flower remedy of all, being a mixture of several different ingredients, namely Star of Bethlehem, Impatiens, Cherry, Plum, Clematis and Rock Rose. It is designed for people in emotional crises, for patients who feel shocked, out of control, mentally numb or in turmoil and panic. It is therefore used by all kinds of different people, from the unemployed through to busy housewives or company executives, and is used as a calming treatment for such diverse problems as exam stress, fear of heights and panic attacks.

Are the remedies effective?

Since scientific analysis of flower remedies can find no trace of the original ingredients, merely detecting the brandy and the spring water, it is easy to assume they work by their placebo effect alone. Certainly no randomized clinical trials have substantiated their therapeutic claims, although anecdotal evidence from many a satisfied customer suggests that they do have an important part to play in treatment, and many medically qualified physicians use them as an adjunct to their own orthodox practices.

What form might the treatment take?

Although there are a few Bach flower therapists who use the remedies entirely on their own, many other complementary therapists combine them with their other work in, for example, aromatherapy, naturopathy or crystal therapy. It is possible to self-administer the remedies, too, but it is usual to obtain guidance, at least initially, as to which remedies to take by consulting an experienced practitioner, who can advise on which remedy would best suit the patient's particular emotional state at the time. To try to discover a patient's true personality, the therapist might ask about their childhood, their experiences as they grew up and attended school, how many friends they have and if they find it easy to make new ones, exploring at the same time their current relationships. He or she might also want to find out how patients react to adverse events in their lives, especially those which register high on the stress scale, such as bereavement, injury, redundancy, or separation. The initial consultation might last for anything between 15 minutes and an hour and a half, and then at the end the therapist would probably suggest a combination of suitable remedies, the final number adding up to maybe half a dozen individual remedies.

Some patients gain immediate beneficial effect from Bach flower remedies, but others with more complicated problems may want to revisit the therapist on several more occasions. Finally, some people find they develop physical or emotional reactions while taking a course of treatment. The therapist would regard this as a positive and helpful sign that negative and damaging emotions are being effectively exorcised.

What problems are helped by Bach flower remedies?

Bach flower remedies are really designed to help people to overcome psychological difficulties and emotional sources of stress. Anxiety, depression, loneliness, grief and bereavement are all commonly treated in this way, and not only can individual adults benefit, but children and animals can enjoy this therapy as well.

Are they safe?

Being so simple and gentle, Bach flower remedies are neither harmful nor addictive and do not interact with any other form of therapy. They can be taken at any age, and for people with any ailment.

How can I find a Bach flower therapist?

The Bach Centre keeps a register of 350 or so therapists, all of whom have successfully completed its three-stage course and have subscribed to a code of practice and ethics. It is possible to obtain free telephone advice from the Centre.

How much will it cost?

A consultation with a Bach Centre practitioner will cost somewhere in the region of £20, and a 10 ml bottle of Rescue Remedy bought off the shelf will cost about £3. In fact, all 38 of the stock flower remedies are available in 10 ml bottles for about the same price.

The sceptic's view

The sceptic might consider Bach flower remedies to be part of every hippy's charter. Gentle to the point of being ineffectual, and natural to the point of being purely botanical, these diluted flower essences can only have a placebo effect. There is nothing of the original flower detectable in the diluent, and the only active ingredient is the alcohol itself. It is quaint to believe that the Impatiens flower can be used to placate impatience, but also somewhat naive. As for giving it safely to animals and children, should children really be given any alcohol at all? When all is said and done, however, flowers do give people joy, and they do blossom through the life-giving energy of the sun, so the sceptic is prepared to tolerate these naturalistic products with a sympathetic level of critical restraint.

The therapist's view

'I have used Bach flower remedies in my practice for many years, and the results have been excellent. The remedies are safe and not addictive; they are not drugs and can be taken alongside other forms of medication without interfering with them in any way.

'There are 38 remedies in all, covering every emotion and state of mind known to humanity. They treat the person not the disease. Star of Bethlehem has given comfort to countless people suffering bereavement; Larch is ideal for someone who has lost self-confidence; Crab apple is a cleansing remedy for those who have skin diseases and feel unclean for any reason. These are but a few of the remedies which have brought comfort and relief to so many people. They can safely be given to children, babies and animals.

'A counselling session lasts about one hour. Up to six or seven remedies can be prescribed in a 30 ml treatment bottle.'

Barbara Stanhope-Williamson, MAR, BRCP

The patient's view

'I was a heroin user for three years. As a result my health suffered, I had low self-esteem, a gaunt look about me, broke out into an uncontrollable rash, *and* I was menopausal, in fact rock-bottom.

'Then I found Barbara and her wonderful Bach flowers, and she instantly put me on a mixture of flower drops. Crab apple was particularly effective. It helped my self-hatred, and, when mixed with Rescue Remedy cream, and rubbed on the skin, it soothed the itching.

'For two years now, Bach flower remedies have lifted me from depression, anger and bad temper, and have helped me to generally feel better about my being.

'Thank you Dr Bach, thank you Barbara.'

Vega John

Chinese Herbal Medicine

(see also Herbal Medicine)

Origins

Like acupuncture, Chinese herbal medicine is part of traditional Chinese medicine and has been practised for over 5,000 years in its Eastern homeland. In fact, these two branches of Chinese philosophy are regarded as complementary opposites, acupuncture representing Yang, since it works from the outside in, and herbalism representing Yin since it works from the inside out.

The earliest major work on Chinese herbal medicine was apparently compiled by Emperor Yen in around 1,500 BC, but collective wisdom on the subject was condensed and refined into a medical text in about AD 200, listing 365 herbs and establishing the basis of Chinese pharmacology. Further experimentation and experience over the years resulted in the publication of Li Shi Zheng's *Beng Cao Gang Mu* (general catalogue of herbs), which was published in the sixteenth century, an impressive collection of tomes which still remains highly regarded today.

In Britain, Chinese herbal medicine has become established wherever a local Chinese community has flourished, and, from the late 1980s onwards, the herbs on which it is based have become increasingly available. It currently represents one of the fastest expanding complementary therapies in the UK, and there are some 260 registered Chinese herbalists practising, between them handing out over one million prescriptions a year.

What is Chinese herbal medicine?

In a nutshell, this is a form of traditional Chinese medicine which employs the properties of a variety of herbs to prevent and treat physical, mental and emotional ill-health. It may be used alone, as it often is in China, or in conjunction with other therapies, such as acupunture or shiatsu, depending on the practitioner and the nature of the patient's complaint. For those patients who are attracted to a gentler form of treatment, or are wary of needles, herbal medicine offers a valuable alternative to acupuncture. Once the practitioner of Chinese herbal medicine has made a diagnosis through traditional methods, herbs are carefully selected to restore balance and harmony to the physical, mental and emotional forces within the patient's body. These herbs are imported into this country from China and Taiwan, and displayed in and dispensed from Chinese pharmacies.

How does it work?

To thoroughly understand Chinese herbal medicine, you need to have a basic knowledge of its underlying philosophy. The Chinese believe that our general state of health depends on our vital energy or 'Chi', and that our 'Xue', or blood, must circulate without restriction at the correct force throughout the body for optimal well-being. They believe that if there is any imbalance or disharmony in the two opposing forces within the Chi (the Yin and Yang) or along the channels through which Xue flows, disease or illness will result. The Chinese philosophy maintains that when Chi flows freely around our body, along the meridians, the Yin and Yang, and the patient as a whole, are in balance and in perfect health. When the energy flow becomes restricted or stagnant and balance is lost, however, illness can result. Chi flows through the 12 major meridians of the body, and interruptions to the energy flow within them can cause problems in corresponding organs. A Chinese herbalist tries to detect any such energy disturbances through his various diagnostic techniques, and then tries to restore the energy balance in the body through the use of specific herbs. He chooses herbs based on their particular attributes and their likely ability to correct disharmony in the body.

Herbs are thought to have one of five different flavours, namely sweet, sour, bitter, salty or pungent. They also possess five Chi attributes (hot, cold, warm, cool or neutral) and four 'directions' (ascending, descending, floating or sinking). According to these attributes herbs are selected to correct the specific imbalance which has been found to exist in the patient's body. For example, if a condition has been diagnosed under that Yin and Yang system and thought to be caused by an energy deficiency, a herb with a toning attribute might be used, whereas a disorder labelled as 'cold' might be treated with a herb noted for its ability to apply warmth. Seeds and roots are more likely to possess descending or sinking inclinations, and might be selected to reduce a person's Chi, and leaves and flowers are more likely to have ascending or floating inclinations and might be selected to raise energy levels and counteract disorders coming from any external source.

Is it effective?

One of the reasons why Chinese herbal medicine appears to be growing so fast in the West is its efficacy in treating certain types of medical disease. This has been shown spectacularly to be the case in the treatment of severe eczema and related skin conditions, which even the most powerful orthodox medicines have sometimes failed to improve. In fact, a carefully designed scientific research study conducted in 1992 has proved without doubt that this gentle treatment is of enormous benefit to eczematous children. The story is fascinating. Children with chronic severe eczema who had been attending Great Ormond Street Hospital for Sick Children in London, but whose eczema had failed to improve despite the use of strong topical steroid creams and applications, and in whom doctors were concerned there might be side effects from such treatment, suddenly began to get dramatically better. What had happened was that these children had been seen by a well-known Chinese herbalist doctor, Dr Luo, in her little shop in Soho, where she had prescribed a decoction of 10 or 12 Chinese herbs all mixed up in a liquorice-flavoured tea.

Although sceptical, the orthodox scientifically trained paediatric skin specialists set about organizing a beautifully designed clinical trial to establish the real efficacy of the herbs. To some children they gave the Chinese herbal tea, and to another group they gave a 'sham' tea (containing no herbal ingredients) and the children were asked to take the treatment for two weeks, followed by a wash-out period of one week, when the children drank neither tea. The children who had been taking the Chinese herbal tea were then given the 'sham' tea, and the children who had been taking the 'sham' tea were given the herbal tea. Both groups were asked to continue the treatment for a further two weeks. When the results were analysed, there was no doubt that all the children's eczema dramatically improved when they were taking the genuine herbal tea, but that when they took the 'sham' tea it remained the same or became worse. Of additional interest was the fact that no obvious side effects were experienced, and adults responded just as the children had in further experiments.

While the Chinese herbalists were not particularly surprised to be shown scientific proof of the efficacy of a treatment they had believed in throughout their lives, the orthodox doctors certainly were surprised by the results, and immediately set about investigating which particular active ingredient amongst the 10 or 12 herbs might be responsible for the amazing clinical improvements. This work continues, and although we still may not know exactly why Chinese herbal tea works for eczema, we do know that it does, and since many orthodox medicines are prescribed with no explicable rationale except that they work, perhaps Chinese herbal medicine will be embraced more readily in the future by conventionally trained members of the medical profession.

What form might the treatment take?

The Chinese herbalist's consulting room might be a separate office, or it might be part of a herbal dispensary which might also be equipped for the provision of acupuncture. The initial consultation for diagnosis will be similar to that used by traditional Chinese acupuncturists, with the proviso that undressing is not necessary. The first and longest consultation lasts for anything up to an hour or so, and during it patients are asked about their lifestyle, diet, exercise, how they feel in themselves, whether they are a calm or anxious person at heart, and, of course, about their current symptoms, their own medical history and their family's medical history. The herbalist will then look at the patient's general appearance, build, weight, and posture, paying particular attention to the face, eyes and tongue. The herbalist will also listen to the patient's voice, breathing patterns and any cough they may have, and of course, test the three pulse positions at each wrist. The herbalist is looking here for 28 different pulse qualities, all of which relate to individual problems. In Chinese medicine, a 'sinking' pulse may be regarded as an indication of internal disharmony, whereas a 'large' pulse might suggest an excess of 'heat' in the stomach.

Having reached a diagnosis, which may or may not occur at the first consultation, the patient might be given a pack of herbs containing mixtures of leaves, seeds and bark or stems, although occasionally ready-made pills or concentrated herbal powders may be prescribed. The herbs will be tailored to the patient's individual needs, and the dose strength will depend on the severity of the problems needing treatment and the patient's health and age. The patient is told how to make up the herbal medicines in water, and whether or not to soak the herbs in water before boiling. Once the boiling has been carried out, the tea should be drunk at various intervals, according to the instructions given. The tea is usually drunk on an empty stomach. The herbalist will usually want to see the patient again a week or so after starting treatment. Depending on the condition being treated, improvement may be quite dramatic, as in, for example, those patients with eczema or insomnia, but for patients with long-standing and serious problems the herbalist will probably recommend regular treatment over a period of many years.

What problems are helped by Chinese herbal medicine?

While Chinese herbal medicine is particularly good at treating skin diseases, especially eczema, it is also of noted benefit for burns, colds, flu, coughs and bronchitis, digestive complaints, certain kinds of asthma, and menstrual irregularities. The World Health Organization has published a list of problems which herbalism can improve, and these include ME (myalgic encephalomyelitis), allergic rhinitis, arthritis, depression, hay fever, infertility, sciatica, pre-menstrual syndrome, insomnia, and even such intractable problems as strokes, diabetes and cerebral palsy. In various parts of the world, Chinese herbalism is also used to boost immunity in order to delay progression of infections such as hepatitis A and B, and AIDS.

Is it safe?

One would imagine that Chinese herbal medicine would be harmless, but this may not necessarily be the case. Provided the herbs are obtained from an importer or supplier with quality controls in place, and are prescribed by a practitioner who is on the register of Chinese Herbal Medicine (RCHM), you should not encounter any difficulties. However, there are risks involved if unqualified and untrained practitioners prescribe inappropriate herbs, or if adequately tráined practitioners prescribe herbs which are contaminated, adulterated or mixed with pharmaceutical drug products or other substances.

The medical toxicology unit at Guy's and St Thomas's Hospital are still monitoring the effect on the liver of certain Chinese herbs after two patients, who were taking herbal medicine for skin disorders, died from liver failure. The RCHM has gone so far as to advise its practitioners to take blood in order to test their patients' liver function prior to treatment, as a precaution. Furthermore, in 1992 in Belgium, a mix-up in supplies meant that a Chinese herbal slimming formulation caused kidney failure in 70 young women, some of whom were tragically left with permanent kidney damage.

The moral is that even something as benign-sounding as Chinese herbs can sometimes have serious side effects and, bearing in mind that some three and a half thousand different herbs, herbal pills and preparations are imported into the UK, it is important that certain safeguards are put in place. Bear in mind that only two members of the Chinese Herbal Suppliers Association exercise regulated quality control of their products. Remember, too, that herbal medicines, whether originating in the West or the East, do not have to be licensed under Section 12 of the Medicines Act 1968 if they are made or supplied by a therapist in a face-to-face consultation. The herbalist doesn't have to identify the ingredients, but the efficacy and safety of what he gives the patient remain entirely his or her responsibility. The patient risks being given something that is fake (recent surveys suggest that about 10 per cent of herbal treatments are not authentic), that may be of substandard quality or that may be contaminated. Also bear in mind that some remedies may contain products derived from endangered species, including tiger bone, rhino horn and other such exotica. If you are taking any kind of Chinese herbal medicine, buy it from a reputable company and ask for precise directions about using the herbs. Make sure you know how to prepare them, and how best to store them. If you should feel unwell, tell the herbalist who prescribed them straight away, and if your symptoms are thought to be due to side effects, the correct procedure is to report these to the Medicines Control Agency so that information can be gathered with a view to protecting other members of the community in the future.

How can I find a Chinese herbal therapist?

In Britain, the title of 'doctor' can only be used by medically qualified professionals who are registered with the General Medical Council, and it is illegal to do so otherwise. There are obviously a few orthodox doctors who are also practitioners of Chinese herbal medicine, but these are few and far between. Most Chinese herbal practitioners receive some training in order to diagnose and treat people with herbs, while herbal pharmacists can dispense herbs but are not registered to practise herbal medicine itself. The trouble is that absolutely anybody can obtain herbs, set up a business and dispense these remedies to unsuspecting clients, and in the UK this is increasingly tending to happen. On the other hand, there are practitioners who have had a full and thorough training in China and are highly skilled in their art. Reputable practitioners tend to be concentrated in Chinatowns, such as London's Soho, but there is no failsafe way to find a good practitioner with the certain knowledge that he or she is safe and effective. I would recommend choosing a practitioner who belongs to the RCHM as all of its members have at least a minimum of five years' training, including three years in traditional orthodox medicine. Registered practitioners follow the RCHM's regulated code of practice and ethics. Only when further compulsory registration of herbal practitioners occurs will this form of Eastern medicine be fully accepted. Furthermore, a crop of highly commercial clinics are springing up which claim to specialize in certain problems, such as skin disorders and stress-related conditions. Such clinics may need to be regarded with some suspicion since one of the founding principles of Chinese herbal medicine is that it is a holistic therapy dealing with the whole person, their mind, body and spirit, rather than just dealing with a collection of individual disorders in one-off consultations lasting just a few minutes.

How much will it cost?

The usual cost of one consultation in this form of complementary therapy is in the region of £25, which does not include the cost of the herbs, ready-made pills or powdered preparations.

The sceptic's view

It is hard for the disbeliever to accept a diagnosis along the lines of 'bladder Yang deficiency with exterior heat in the triple warmer meridian' without a degree of bemusement. However, although he or she might scoff at the ability of the Chinese herbalist to distinguish between 28 different pulse qualities, and to locate signs of energy blockages along invisible meridians in the body, the sceptic would have to acknowledge that at least in the field of eczema Chinese herbal concoctions have proved to be of real and significant scientific value. They have succeeded where even the most potent orthodox preparations, including steroids, have failed, even when they were used in sufficiently high dosage to cause worrying side effects in their own right. The sceptic would, however, be alarmed at the lack of regulation of the majority of Chinese herbalists in this country, and at the fact that so far only two of the various importers and suppliers of herbs in Britain exercise any meaningful level of quality control on their products. Chinese herbs may be subject to contamination, adulteration, and may not even be authentic; they can contain traces of heavy metals and other toxic substances, and, quite apart from anything else, they might consist partly of the ground-up by-products of endangered species, including rhino and tiger. The entrenched sceptic is likely to want to know how many untrained practitioners of Chinese herbal medicine have failed to make a proper diagnosis of a serious condition, and whose delay in failing to encourage their client to seek conventional help has resulted in a potentially curable condition becoming incurable.

The therapist's view

The practitioner would claim that the popularity and rapid growth of Chinese herbal medicine speaks for itself. It is a satisfying and gentle form of therapy, using natural products combined with specific skills in diagnosis and the selection of individual herbs. It is a holistic therapy, calling upon the ancient Chinese philosophies and incorporating all elements of mind, body and spirit. It may be practised along with acupuncture, although not necessarily, and well-designed scientific trials have shown the treatment to be of great value in the treatment of both children and adults, particularly in the area of skin problems.

The patient's view

'I'd always had bad eczema and for years I'd had to put bandages on at night to keep my skin moist and stop me from scratching. Sometimes the eczema

would get infected and I'd have to use lots of antibiotics. Kids at school used to call me the leper because it looked so awful but I certainly didn't find it funny. The doctors always said I'd grow out of it and that they couldn't give me treatment that was too strong because of the side effects it might have. What they did give me though didn't seem very helpful, although they must have given me hundreds of things. My dad seemed more concerned about my eczema than I did, I think, and eventually he took me up to a place in Chinatown in London where this Chinese doctor gave me a special herbal tea mixed with liquorice. It tasted horrible, but it was worth it as two weeks later my skin was almost clear. My doctor checked my blood to make sure my liver wasn't affected by the tea, and it wasn't, and I'm still taking it. My dad thinks it's a miracle, and I have to agree. I'm very grateful to the doctor, and perhaps I'll go and live in China when I'm older.'

Mark Devene (aged 9)

Chiropractic

Origins

The name 'chiropractic' comes from two Greek words – *praktikos*, meaning 'performed by', and *cheir*, meaning 'hand'. Physical manipulation of the spine was almost certainly carried out thousands of years ago by the ancient Greeks and the Chinese, and in the Middle Ages 'bone-setters' were often called upon to correct dislocations and realign all kinds of muscular and skeletal disorders ranging from soft tissue inflammations to serious compound fractures. However, modern chiropractic therapy, as it is now known, was founded in 1895 by a Canadian osteopath and magnetic healer by the name of Daniel David Palmer. The story goes that he cured his office janitor, Harvey Lillard, of long-standing deafness which the patient always claimed had begun when something clicked in his back. Palmer apparently manipulated the badly aligned vertebrae and the janitor's hearing recovered. Later he set up the Palmer Infirmary and Chiropractic Institute in Iowa, and now some 20 million Americans are treated with chiropractic each year. The British Chiropractic Association was set up in 1925 and in 1965 the first chiropractic college outside America was opened in Bournemouth, the Anglo-

European College of Chiropractic. Other colleges have since sprung up, notably the McTimoney College and the Oxford College of Chiropractic. There are nearly 1,000 chiropractors working in Britain today.

What is chiropractic?

Basically, chiropractic is a manipulative treatment which concentrates on the musculo-skeletal system, particularly on the spine and nervous system. It is used to relieve non-specific low back pain, shoulder and hip pain, and to relieve problems not usually associated with the spine, such as digestive complaints and asthma. Through detailed physical examination and manipulative therapy, chiropractors attempt to diagnose and correct problems connected with the musculo-skeletal system. These disorders are not necessarily confined to the muscles, ligaments, tendons and nerves in close proximity to the spine, because chiropractors believe that by altering the function of the nervous system generally, the health of the rest of the body can be improved. Everything from headaches, sports injuries, sciatica, hip pain and fibrositis can therefore benefit.

How does it work?

By using their hands, the chiropractors aim to manipulate joints and muscles to relieve pain, to increase the range of movement in a joint and to improve function. In so doing chiropractors hope to reduce stress and improve a patient's posture, as well as counteracting the damaging mechanical forces of gravity on the joints, and putting right any damage incurred through previous trauma. Unlike osteopaths, who often work on several joints at once, using the limbs as levers, chiropractors tend to work on one joint at a time. They are more likely to use X-rays to reach their diagnosis, and chiropractic manipulation is largely confined to the spine. By restoring full structural integrity to the spine, the aim of chiropractic therapy is to promote homeostasis (the biological status quo) within the nervous system from which all other organs in the body will benefit.

Different chiropractic techniques may be employed, which aim to take an individual joint just beyond its normal range of active movement to stretch it, realign it or break down the fibrous adhesions. Soft tissue techniques help reduce any muscle spasm and encourage the patient to relax before manipulation begins. Trigger points may be massaged and relief may follow in much the same way as it does through massage carried out on the acupressure points referred to in traditional Chinese medicine. 'Direct thrust' techniques are quick and vigorous movements, delivered at speed to adjust the alignment and position of the joint. Cracking noises may be heard as this happens. representing the rupture of tiny gas bubbles in the synovial fluid which exists between all synovial joint surfaces. For some patients, these techniques are unpleasant, so the less forceful 'indirect thrust' technique is used. Here, the joint is more gradually and gently extended over a supportive pad or towel.

Is chiropractic effective?

In 1995 the Medical Research Council conducted a scientific study comparing chiropractic with conventional hospital treatment for low back pain. Continued over three years, the findings weighed heavily in favour of chiropractic because the improvement in pain relief was nearly 30 per cent greater in the patients treated with chiropractic than in those referred to hospital out-patient departments in the usual way. In addition, five years later, the patients treated with chiropractic were still 20 per cent better off than the group treated by orthodox means. Other studies have also found very much in favour of chiropractic techniques, and in view of the startling statistics regarding the current epidemic of low back pain in Britain, its potential benefits and applications should not be underestimated.

The National Back Pain Association regards back pain as the

single most important cause of absenteeism from work, with some 120 million working days lost every year. This is an economically devastating statistic as the cost to the NHS approaches nearly £100 million annually. Chiropractic is both cheaper and potentially more available than hospital out-patient treatment and it is particularly effective when used for acute back ache in order to prevent chronic problems setting in. If chiropractic were used more routinely, the potential savings for the NHS would be huge.

What form might the treatment take?

At the first consultation, which will last for 30 minutes to an hour, the usual medical history is taken and a physical examination carried out. The therapist attempts to learn as much as possible about the patient, enquiring about their lifestyle, their level of physical activity, their outlook and personality, their occupation and their social lives. Once a thorough examination has been carried out, samples of blood or urine may be required. X-rays may or may not be taken, but most chiropractors have their own X-ray facilities and frequently use them. This is important since not only can X-rays confirm what is found through clinical examination, but they can sometimes reveal undiagnosed disease for which manipulative treatment would be counter-productive or even dangerous. If this kind of problem is discovered the chiropractor will refer the patient back to their GP for more appropriate investigation and treatment.

Chiropractic treatment is often delayed until the second appointment as the history and physical examination will take up the majority of the first consultation. Various techniques may be used, but the first step might be to apply soft tissue manipulation to relax points of tenderness and to dissipate tension in any trigger points. Other forms of manipulation, such as the 'direct' and 'indirect thrust' techniques above are then used, with the patient either sitting or lying down on a special couch. Each time a direct or indirect thrust technique is employed, the force is sudden and momentary and over in a fraction of a second. The cracking noises from the joint are quite normal.

The number of sessions the patient needs depends entirely on the cause of the problem and how they respond to treatment. A simple alignment of a single joint in the neck may only require one treatment, but more chronic conditions or disorders arising from malalignment of several parts of the spine may require up to a dozen treatments over a period of 2–3 months. Problems like frozen shoulder, which arise insidiously and which progressively become more severe, may take even longer to correct. In addition to being manipulated, the patient is generally given advice on their overall posture and how to rest correctly, what they should be eating and how they should be exercising. This is important because some rheumatic conditions require rest, while others require mobilization.

What problems are helped by chiropractic?

There is no doubt that all back-related problems, whether they are in the neck, the shoulder blades or in the lower part of the spine, form the bulk of the chiropractor's workload. However, shoulder problems, tension headaches, migraines, tennis elbow, hip pain, immobility or ankle injury also commonly fall within the realms of chiropractic techniques. In addition, digestive disorders, menstrual disorders, asthma, irritable bowel syndrome and constipation may all respond to this kind of therapy.

Is it safe?

Where there is systemic disease affecting bones, as in leukaemia or multiple myeloma, for instance, where bone is eroded by malignant deposits, and in osteoporosis (brittle bone disease), chiropractic therapy is not suitable. This is why the first consultation with the chiropractor is so important: the patient's detailed history, their physical examination and other investigations, particularly X-rays, are analysed to rule these conditions out prior to any manipulation.

Generally speaking, however, provided the chiropractor is qualified and properly registered, the technique is safe for all age groups, including new-born babies, pregnant women and the elderly, though, of course, X-rays should never be used in pregnancy without very careful consideration.

How can I find a chiropractor?

GPs are more used to referring their NHS patients with musculo-skeletal disorders to physiotherapists whose services are available free of charge under the NHS, but there is nothing to prevent a GP from referring a patient to a chiropractor, and in fact, this is increasingly likely to happen these days. GP fundholders may even be able to finance chiropractic treatment by diverting their NHS funds for this purpose. A study conducted by the Department of Health in 1996 started a pilot project amongst fundholding practices to look into this very possibility, and, later the same year, the Royal College of General Practitioners issued guidelines to family doctors specifically recommending manipulative therapy rather than other treatments for patients with back pain within the first six weeks of their disorder.

Since most patients still have to see chiropractors privately, however, they need to know who to approach. Often the GP can recommend somebody he or she knows and trusts locally. If not, find a practitioner registered with the British Chiropractic Association, the Scottish Chiropractic Association, the McTimoney Chiropractic Association or the British Association for Applied Chiropractic. The training afforded by these different groups varies but under the Chiropractic Act of 1994, it is hoped that the General Chiropractic Council will regulate all branches of the profession in an attempt to maintain and guarantee proper standards of training and competence among registered members.

Chiropractic is one of the most popular complementary therapies of all, with a high reported level of satisfaction in terms of symptom relief. After osteopathy, it is the second complementary therapy to have legally regulated itself, and this has encouraged the orthodox medical profession to embrace its undoubted therapeutic application more warmly.

How much will it cost?

You can expect to pay anywhere between £20 and £40 for the first consultation, but subsequent sessions might be £5–10 less.

The sceptic's view

Even the most die-hard sceptic would have to accept, albeit grudgingly, that chiropractic has proved its worth when compared to orthodox medical practices used in the treatment of low back pain. Many an orthodox doctor has been made to feel slightly uncomfortable when one of their own registered patients, who has failed to respond to any of the prescribed treatments supplied by themselves over a long period of time, returns after a first visit to the chiropractor, marvelling at the response they have had and to telling the doctor how much they wish they had been before. The sceptic has to accept, therefore, that chiropractic has a place, but he or she is not able to agree that by manipulating the spine a patient's digestive problems or asthma can be improved. This does not fall within any anatomical or physiological parameters in which the orthodox doctor has been trained, and the sceptic would not be able to concur either with the chiropractor that his training is every bit as detailed and comprehensive as that of the orthodox doctor. Chiropractors may well be able to carry out their own X-rays, blood and urine tests, but are they really as far-reaching and conclusive as those carried out in an NHS trust hospital?

The therapist's view

'Historically, the "art" of chiropractic allowed successful development of techniques for treating people with a conceptual understanding of "diagnosis" leading to the adoption of such terms as the "subluxation" (mechanism of "dis-ease" in the joint) and the "innate" (a lift-force governing wellness). The "science" has been used to try and explain the "art" and more recently to consider relevant ways of measuring and increasing the effectiveness of chiropractic giving us "evidence-based" practice.

'The general public is now much more enquiring about its health care. Patients frequently complain that while they accept the system of labelling, e. g. "sciatica", "lumbago" and "arthritis", they do not understand what those terms actually mean and to what extent they apply to them. Of course, chiropractic effectively treats those conditions along with more specifically labelled problems such as "trapped nerve", "torticollis" and "migraine", but it is the chiropractor's emphasis on helping patients to understand their problems that gives them the opportunity to help themselves.

'In a recent sample of my practice, 299 out of 500 patients (60 per cent) did not know why their problem started, emphasizing the importance of considering that problem in the context of their normal lives. I will make a diagnosis of a patient's problem, explain it to them, and then we will work together. My role is clearly treatment, but I must also manage the patient, constantly monitoring feedback to consider all environmental factors. This balance of correct diagnosis and treatment with management of work and lifestyle problems enables me to achieve a high rate of successful outcome and the patient to reduce likelihood of recurrence.'

Gordon K. Linscott, DC

The patient's view

'I worked as a PA in a busy computer firm and spent a lot of my time sitting at a desk working a computer keyboard. I often experienced aching shoulders and tension headaches as a result of neck strain, and on more than one occasion I had long absences from work with repetitive strain injury (RSI). My doctor used to give me anti-inflammatory tablets for my neck trouble, claiming that the strain was the result of an old neck injury I sustained in a car accident. Eventually I consulted a chiropractor who within a week had rendered me completely pain free. The massage and manipulation techniques he used were comfortable and the freedom of movement he achieved in my entire spine I could hardly believe. He also taught me exercises to prevent further strain occurring in my deskbound job, and in the two years since I first saw him, I have not experienced any further trouble.'

Dana Morgan

Colonic Hydrotherapy

Origins

Purging, through the use of enemas, was practised by the ancient Egyptians and Chinese, and has been used ever since in many countries throughout the world. In Britain, in the earlier part of this century, regular enemas were generally considered beneficial, and 'colon laundries' were even set up in London with the aim of ridding people of their ailments. In the last decade, colonic hydrotherapy, or colonic irrigation as it is more often called, has again become reasonably fashionable, particularly amongst the 'worried well' of the aristocracy and upper middle classes.

What is colonic hydrotherapy?

Colonic hydrotherapy is known by the French as *lavage*, and involves washing out the large intestine in an effort to improve the patient's health. The fundamental principle is that the colon becomes unhealthy when it becomes contaminated by toxins and the overgrowth of unwelcome bacteria. When these are combined with faecal material, mucus and digestive secretions, the intestine can only function at suboptimal levels, producing a variety of symptoms elsewhere in the body. The lower intestinal tract is uniquely associated with human waste disposal in the minds of most people, so the idea that its functional stagnation can produce ill-health is hugely appealing to many. For those people brought up and conditioned to believe that anything to do with bowels and intestinal physiology is 'dirty' and best not mentioned, the thought of having the whole system washed out is logical and welcome. Only the thought of how it might be done inhibits them.

How does it work?

Colonic irrigation aims to eradicate harmful bacteria from the gut and to flush out any toxins lurking there. Its intention is to 'spring-clean' the lining of the bowel, removing deposits of mucus, which are secreted from the cells in its walls, and to dispel the effect of any malodorous gases and faecal matter hiding in the various crypts and recesses along its length. It involves the replacement of unwelcome bacteria with healthier varieties, such as *lactobacilli*, which are better able to combat thrush organisms and stimulate improved function. It is widely believed to be of particular benefit to patients prone to constipation, especially those who suffer occasional abdominal discomfort as a result of flatulence.

Is colonic hydrotherapy effective?

As a form of enema, colonic hydrotherapy may be of benefit to people whose constipation is resistant to more conventional treatment, including the use of laxatives, but there is no evidence that it improves bowel function, nor that people willing to have it done have any gastrointestinal abnormalities in the first place. One of the main functions of the colon is to excrete waste products while at the same time reabsorbing water in order to achieve proper mineral and water balance within the body. Its wall is designed to act as a selective filter in this way, and as such it is already extremely efficient. Any toxins found within the lumen (the hollow passage that runs along the length of the colon) have every right to be there, as have the bacteria which achieve a useful biological balance in normal circumstances. Consultant gastroenterologists are generally horrified at the thought of interfering by washing out the very things that Mother Nature put there. Mucus production by the cells within the colon provides lubrication of the intestinal lining so that food residues can pass smoothly through it. Water absorption proceeds according to the state of hydration in the body and the food residue content of the bowel. Removing the normal bacterial flora and interfering with the subtle balance of biological tasks carried out by the colon is theoretically harmful. Furthermore, any attempt to replace these normal bacteria with *lactobacillus acidophilus*, given in the form of a drink, has not been shown to be of significant value in any medical condition. All in all, colonic hydrotherapy may well help those people who have been brought up to believe their bowels are filthy and require a thorough cleaning but there is no scientific evidence whatsoever to show that it can benefit any physical condition, except perhaps intractable constipation.

What form might the treatment take?

When seeing a colonic hydrotherapist, the patient's medical history will be investigated, and the practical procedure of colonic irrigation explained. The patient strips off and puts on a gown, and then lies on their side on a couch or table so that a lubricated sterile speculum can be inserted into the anus. Next, while the patient lies on their back with their knees bent at right angles, water is pumped into the large intestine at low pressure through a narrow sterile tube. Once the water has all been pumped in, it is then drawn out again through a separate tube, the whole cycle taking about 45 minutes. The patient later releases any remaining water into the lavatory and is asked to take a drink containing *lactobacillus acidophilus* bacteria in the hope that it will colonize the cleaned colon. The whole procedure is generally not uncomfortable and some patients even notice an immediate improvement in the way they feel. Some therapists recommend that patients have a regular course of several sessions at fortnightly intervals, at least to begin with, and many patients take up the offer. Other patients, however, seem happy to have an occasional treatment once or twice a year, often depending on how they feel about themselves at the time.

What problems are helped by colonic hydrotherapy?

Whilst not as good as a medicinal laxative enema, colonic hydrotherapy can certainly wash out colonic contents. Whether this is in any way beneficial or not is controversial. Some therapists claim that regular colonic irrigation can improve the lustre of the skin, stimulate the circulation, help in losing weight and reduce headaches. It is also used to alleviate depression, and offers hope to people written off by the medical profession, including people suffering from ME (myalgic encephalomyelitis) or irritable bowel syndrome (IBS). In fact, one of the reasons why colonic hydrotherapy has gained favour in some sections of society is that amongst the seven million people who currently suffer with IBS and have to put up with alternating diarrhoea and constipation, wind and flatutence, abdominal cramps and bloating, many feel let down and dismissed by orthodox practitioners. They are told that their symptoms are due to stress and worry, and the implication is that they are neurotic. Since twice as many women as men are affected, and since women are more adventurous in trying alternative therapies, it is no wonder that many turn to colonic irrigation, at least as a harmless experiment. Some 20 million laxatives a year are used in Britain by those who have been brainwashed into believing that they must have a bowel action every day to be healthy, and colonic hydrotherapy has flourished in recent times partly as a result of these 20 million being advised that overuse of laxatives is harmful as it encourages a lazy bowel or spastic colon. Colonic hydrotherapy is therefore used by IBS sufferers, particularly in conjunction with other forms of complementary therapy.

Is it safe?

The greatest risk of colonic irrigation, or *lavage*, is perforation of the colon by the tube which is inserted. Whilst the water is only pumped into the bowel under low pressure, and only the bluntest of tubes is gently inserted, perforation of any hollow organ in the body is a recognized complication of any invasive technique. Furthermore, the irrigation of the intestine with significant volumes of water is potentially enough to unbalance the body's salt and water ratio. The procedure temporarily alters the flora of micro-organisms inhabiting the bowel, but this is almost certainly not enough to cause any lasting harm.

How can I find a colonic hydrotherapist?

Insist on going to somebody who is a member of the Colonic International Association. This is not a therapy that one would want to endure if the therapist were an unregistered beginner. Members of the CIA have their premises inspected at regular intervals and are obliged to attend refresher courses annually.

How much will it cost?

The cost of treatment varies between £35 and £55, depending on the area of the country in which your chosen therapist works.

The sceptic's view

The sceptic might view colonic hydrotherapy as the ideal treatment for neurotics who remain stubbornly anally retentive. With a fixation about their bowels and the motions that emerge from them, these people can only think in concrete terms, and the only way out of their psychological obsession is a physical washout. It is a kind of obsessional compulsive behaviour in someone who has a phobia about their own intestines.

The therapist's view

'A few doctors refer patients to me but sadly most of them view colonics as merely a "wash out". For many people, attention to bowel dysfunction early in life could very well make the difference between longevity and a tragically shortened lifespan. It is most unfortunate that people are so inhibited about the lower end of their alimentary canal. Much skill is required on my part to reassure and relax them. I am often thanked for making the whole experience more pleasant than had been anticipated. Needless to say, I do advise on a healthier diet which includes more fruit, salads and vegetables, adequate pure water, and reduction, if not avoidance of mucoid-forming, nutritionally dead foods. Also helpful is the recommendation of various practices to aid in reducing stress which so directly affects normal bowel function.'

Mary Chase Hopkins

The patient's view

'I had suffered over the years with digestive difficulties, bloating, flatulence, tummy tenderness, pain and constipation, which seemed to get worse over time, and I became very tired, suffered from migraines, low moods, lightheadedness, lack of concentration and lethargy.

'I was diagnosed by a consultant, through my GP, as having IBS [Irritable Bowel Syndrome] and was given a medical bulking agent called isphagula husk, which made me even more bloated and uncomfortable.

'In April 1996 I had a cyst removed from my ovary and after that operation my health deteriorated and I knew I could not go on feeling like this, with such discomfort at times.

'I went to see a naturopath who took me off wheat, yeast, dairy products, sugar, coffee, tea, etc, and I booked a course of colonics over a short period. The combination produced incredible results and I began to feel alive again, my bowel movements became regular, my thinking and sense of well-being were incredible, I was less bloated and my migraines completely stopped.

'Now, I am still careful with my diet and know my limitations. I have colonics occasionally, if I feel the need. I realize just how important elimination is and I would not wish to go back to feeling the way I did.

'The experience of having a colonic was not at all unpleasant for me and I would recommend them to anyone who suffers from digestive difficulties, combined with a suitable diet. Finally, I would recommend anybody considering colonics to find a therapist they feel at ease with. This makes a tremendous difference.'

Jennifer Smith

Colour therapy

Origins

Colour has long been associated with mood, and many Greek or Egyptian temples were adorned with specific colour for its therapeutic effect. Thousands of years ago, the Chinese would wrap people in coloured silk to cure them of certain conditions, and Buddhists are still taught to acknowledge the importance of colour in meditation. Even the stained glass windows in Christian churches were thought to increase the spiritual power of prayer.

What is colour therapy?

Colour therapy is a form of energy medicine which uses the radiation present in all the colours of the visible and invisible spectrum to prevent and treat physical, emotional and psychological ill-health. As such, it is often used in conjunction with other therapies by reflexologists, acupuncturists, aromatherapists and others.

How does it work?

In much the same way that X-rays and the sun's ultraviolet light can influence our health, the vibrating energy of the electromagnetic waves coming from light rays can bring about alterations in our medical status quo. The theory behind colour therapy is that our bodies emit an energy field, or 'aura', which some people claim to see as a haze of coloured light around our bodies, and which reflects all aspects of our being and reveals how we are feeling on a physical and spiritual plain. Colour therapy is designed to alter any cellular disharmony or disequilibrium in the body and to restore it to a normal healthy state. On one level, a client's exposure to certain colours can simply make them feel better, and this is what image consultants and colour psychologists do to try to make the most of your colour sense and personality. In addition, colour therapists claim to be able to alleviate real medical conditions through the use and application of carefully selected colours.

Is colour therapy effective?

Some work has been done in the form of controlled studies to look into the value of colour therapy, and it has been suggested that the discomfort of rheumatoid arthritis and the frequency of migraine could be reduced by exposing patients to certain wavelengths of light. However, no concrete scientific evidence exists to show beyond all doubt that this is truly beneficial.

Colour therapy may certainly lift a person's mood (and the world may look a much more pleasant place through rose-tinted spectacles), but people with serious disease should not be persuaded that their predicament can be alleviated in this way.

What form might the treatment take?

Patients need to allow a couple of hours the first time they see a colour therapist, and be prepared to divulge any symptoms they might be suffering from, and their previous medical history. Patients are likely to be asked about their personality and emotional states and may well be asked to select their favourite colours from a selection of different-coloured cards or balls. Depending on the therapist's methods, one colour will be selected as the mainstay of the patient's treatment, and this will be prescribed along with a complementary colour to increase the healing ability of the first. Colour therapy may come in the form of crystals, light, silk scarves or even coloured water. Coloured light might be applied to the seven chakras, or energy centres, of the body and quite often the therapist will ask the patient to do some work on their own at home, which involves eating foods of a certain colour, visualizing colours at moments throughout the day, and wearing clothes of a particular hue.

What problems are helped by colour therapy?

Claims are made that colour therapy can not only make people feel better generally, but can even help people with serious disorders such as AIDS or cancer. Generally speaking, however, this treatment is used holistically to improve mental, emotional and physical well-being, and to treat stress-related conditions such as insomnia, asthma, behavioural disorders and depression.

Is it safe?

The main problem with colour therapy is that most therapists are not clinically trained, and may be totally unable to diagnose any significant illness. Theoretically, colour therapy should be quite safe, but if it does do what its exponents claim it does, people suffering from conditions like heart disease, high blood pressure and epilepsy could if treated with the wrong choice of light, such as red light, take a turn for the worse, and patients incorrectly treated for hyperactivity with violet light could go off the rails. Patients should always be encouraged to see a conventionally trained doctor before investigating colour therapy.

How can I find a colour therapist?

This form of complementary therapy is totally unregulated, and many a charlatan could happily take your money for the privilege of sitting you under some fancy coloured lighting. A good policy would be to look for a practitioner trained by the International Association for Colour Therapy (IACT), in which case they are likely to have the letters HCertCTh or HDipCTh after their name. Other colour therapists may use the letters IACT and practitioners who have worked for two years or more may apply to be placed on the British Register of Complementary Practitioners.

How much will it cost?

For the first two-hour session, patients can expect to pay around £45 and then £25 for any subsequent consultations. Colour psychologists advising corporate clients may charge more – up to about £80 for the first session, and possibly £40 for further advice.

The sceptic's view

The sceptic might argue that colour therapists are merely tricking patients into parting with their money on the spurious basis that literary language is littered with associations between mood and colour, and that therefore some real link must exist. It is convenient to believe we are under a black cloud if we are depressed, that the red mist comes down when we are angry, that we feel blue when we are lonely or unloved, and that we can be purple with rage or green with envy, but this is infantile and simplistic. We are only black when we are depressed because we stay indoors and don't see the daylight. We are only purple with rage because that's the colour our cheeks go when we are furious. And the idea that a 'specialist colour therapist' can see auric colours surrounding us is too ridiculous for words. We all need to be surrounded by a variety of changing colours and this is both natural and universal. Light therapy in itself has been shown to help people with seasonal affective disorder, but this is diffused light of a mixture of colours, and there is no evidence whatsoever that any one wavelength of light has special healing properties in any individual condition. The idea that the colour turquoise can strengthen the immune system, and that green is beneficial to people with cancer, is both unproven and frankly dangerous. Colour therapy does not work and is often carried out by money-grabbing charlatans making vast sums of money at the expense of gullible victims.

The therapist's view

'People come to see me for a number of reasons. Some are feeling sad or depressed, some find it difficult to control their rages and bad moods, some work in creative employment and complain they have run out of ideas, and some tell me about their physical problems with which no conventional therapist has been able to help them. I spend a generous amount of time with them, often in excess of two hours, and more often than not I am able to see the colour of their aura. To me this is a visible sheen which surrounds their entire body, and from it I can determine which colour they require to reverse any process of disease. I change their auric colours using a combination of coloured light, coloured material and specially chosen make-up. I also advise on interior design in the client's home, and even suggest food of a particular colour chosen for the individual. People are amazed how much colour therapy can lift their mood and make them feel so much more positive about life in general.'

Mary Bennet

The patient's view

' After university I went through a fairly traumatic time in my life and ended up having a nervous breakdown. I had all the conventional treatments that you might expect, including antidepressants and a short course of electro-convulsive therapy which I have to admit was helpful but significantly affected my short-term memory. I continued to have emotional and psychological difficulties, however, and it was suggested I try colour therapy to complement the other treatment I was receiving. The therapist uses specially selected coloured lights which are focused on different parts of my body as I lie there in a white robe. And I also have a special lamp that I can use to flood my bedroom at home with coloured light whenever I'm feeling miserable or tense. I do find it very soothing and, along with my other treatment, I find it works very well for me.'

Patsy Wendle

Cranial Osteopathy

Origins

The fundamental principles of cranial osteopathy have their origins in ordinary osteopathy, as devised by Andrew Taylor Still (see page 268). One of his students, the American William Garland Sutherland, developed a specific type of osteopathy in the 1930s, which he called cranial osteopathy. He came to the conclusion that the skull bones, which develop separately in several different sections in infancy and fuse together to form a rigid continuous shell surrounding the brain in adulthood, could, contrary to orthodox thinking, actually move, and therefore be capable of producing malfunction elsewhere in the body. He argued that by manipulating the skull bones in a very gentle way, the circulation of the cerebro-spinal fluid, which surrounds and protects the brain could be altered. He believed that this fluid possessed 'breath of life rhythms' which influenced human conditions, and that he could balance its flow, thus stimulating the body to heal itself.

What is cranial osteopathy?

This is a specialist osteopathic technique involving such gentle and deft touch that many people subjecting themselves to it are barely aware that it is happening. This particular technique is one of the many indirect techniques that all osteopaths may use at certain times, but by no means all osteopaths use it. Indeed, some general osteopaths frown on its use and do not believe it has a place in modern osteopathy. The technique never uses any significant force, but relies on the very subtle re-positioning of joints and unwinding of soft tissues.

How does it work?

Cranial osteopaths try to alter the rhythm of the cerebro-spinal fluid within and around the brain and surrounding the spinal cord by exerting subtle and gentle pressure on the patient's skull bones. They attempt to manipulate the bones to restore a rhythmic balance to the fluid and as a result correct malfunction in the rest of the body. A cranial osteopath might attribute a sick child's disorder to skull compression caused by a traumatic birth, or to any kind of head injury occurring at a later time. Since the manipulative technique used is so delicate, this form of treatment is often used on children, and indeed has a devoted following amongst parents of children affected by cerebral palsy, autism and mental handicap.

Is cranial osteopathy effective?

Few conventionally trained doctors believe cranial osteopathy is effective, and none recognize the 'cranial rhythmic impulse' that these specialist osteopaths believe exists in the cerebro-spinal fluid. Furthermore, no scientific evidence supports its ability to cure disease. Having said that, many practitioners can supply names of satisfied customers, particularly those of patients who were written off by orthodox doctors as being hopeless cases but whose chronic and disabling symptoms have either improved or become a great deal more bearable as a result of cranial osteopathy.

What form might the treatment take?

The initial consultation will be of about one hour's duration, with subsequent sessions lasting for about half as long. A medical history is taken and a physical examination carried out in much the same way as when consulting any other osteopath, after which the cranial osteopath will focus particularly on the areas of the head and sacral region, where he or she will feel for the 'cranial rhythmic impulse'. The practitioner will then make a diagnosis and put forward a plan of treatment for the future, during which he or she will attempt to rebalance any abnormal rhythm using the gentle pressure technique. Any treatment supplied is gentle and delicate, and most practitioners like to see their patients on a weekly basis. As with general osteopathy, if no improvement is apparent after three or four treatments, a reputable practitioner might consider an alternative approach.

What problems are helped by cranial osteopathy?

The same sort of problems treated by general osteopathy lend themselves to therapy using this technique. It is particularly helpful for babies, and is promoted as being especially useful for adults with sinus problems, temporo-mandibular joint dysfunction, dizziness, tension headache and migraine. It also has a following amongst parents of children with cerebral palsy, autism and other congenital or traumatic problems.

Is it safe?

Like many therapies, cranial osteopathy is not suitable for people with organic mental illness or psychological disturbance, but as it is a physically delicate procedure, it is entirely safe for people of all ages, including newborn babies and the elderly.

How can I find a cranial osteopath?

Make sure that the practitioner you choose is properly trained and fully qualified and registered with a recognized organization (see page 275). Remember that not all osteopaths have undergone training in cranial techniques, and they should not attempt to practise them unless they have. To find a local cranial osteopath who satisfies these criteria send a stamped, self-addressed envelope to the Osteopathic Information Service (OIS), requesting information on cranial osteopathy specifically.

How much will it cost?

The first consultation will cost up to £60–70, with follow-up visits costing about half as much.

The sceptic's view

Cranial osteopathy is patently nonsense because no 'cranial rhythmic impulse' actually exists. Such a notion might be compared with the heart-beat, for example, which sends a wave of pressure through the arteries and is detectable in the neck, groin and wrist. This is palpable and measurable; it is generated by the contraction of the heart. Similarly the lungs expand and contract on breathing, and this is measurable and detectable in the chest wall. But the cerebro-spinal fluid does not pulsate, nor is there any movement of the spinal cord or brain to generate such a pulse. The flow of cerebro-spinal fluid is passive, and affected only marginally by body movement, respiration and strong abdominal contraction. The skull bones do not move either; they are permanently fused together by immovable bridges of bone, and exist in this state from the age of about 18 months at the latest. You cannot manipulate skull bones. If you could, even minor bumps on the head would result in alarmingly dangerous symptoms. Gentle and delicate touching on the head by the cranial osteopath is no more than glorified spiritual healing, and has no place in modern medicine. Of course, there are people who would love to believe that their incurable children are benefiting from such attention, but the sad truth is that they are not, and any apparent improvements are all in the mind. Why is it that no proper scientific studies have been properly carried out to see if this therapy works? Is it because the therapists have something to hide?

The therapist's view

'The cranial osteopathic approach is a satisfying yet highly challenging mode of clinical practice. Mechanical restrictions in joints and soft tissues throughout the body can be responsible for all manner of symptoms, and this applies just as much to restriction of the small tolerances of movement in the sutural joints in the skull as elsewhere. Certain types of conditions, such as tinnitus, dizziness and head pain (such as migraine, trigeminal neuralgia, sinusitis, and temporo-mandibular joint pain), which in many cases have defied other forms of treatment, may be caused by past trauma, and will often respond to the subtle, mechanically based manual treatment methods of the cranial osteopath. This approach can also be used to good effect in the treatment of problems in other areas of the body, including spine and limb pain, particularly when more vigorous treatment should be avoided.

'Some of the most rewarding cases for me are the growing number of children being brought for treatment with complaints that have been caused by a difficult birth. Conditions as diverse as infantile colic, glue ear and poor sleep pattern to delayed development (for example, late walking or speech, or problems with particular areas of schoolwork), and cases of cerebral palsy, often respond well to treatment. Whilst some of them cannot be expected to make a complete recovery, there is no doubt in my mind that the cranial osteopathic approach makes a significant contribution to improving the health and development of these young people.

'An essential feature of osteopathy, whether cranial or otherwise, is the way the practitioner uses a highly refined sense of touch to interpret exactly what treatment is needed in each individual patient at each appointment. The cranial approach, for me, enables me to continually refine these manual skills, as well as constantly striving to improve my diagnostic and clinical management abilities, which means there is always something new to learn.

'One of the frustrations of cranial osteopathic practice is the current lack of valid clinical research to substantiate the results being achieved daily in practices throughout the country. It is my earnest hope that in the near future the osteopathic profession will secure independent support for research into the effectiveness of this approach.'

Nicholas Woodhead, DO
Council Member, General Osteopathic Council

The patient's view

'I am 41 years of age and have suffered from migraine since the age of 15. During the last few years the frequency and intensity of the attacks increased until they were lasting for four days a week for three weeks in the month, and my life was totally unbearable. I could not plan a holiday or a short break without migraine ruining and curtailing it. It also added stress to my working life as in the end I could not even think straight.

'I read about cranial osteopathy in a women's magazine, and decided to give it a try and booked an appointment. The consultation and examination were very thorough and the osteopath's initial suggestion was for me to have an MRI scan as he was concerned about the obvious deterioration in my health. However, before agreeing to have the scan I wanted the osteopath to treat me, although I was desperate and willing to try anything to relieve the misery, I did not raise my hopes. The treatment was very gentle and I was surprised when, following one of the treatments, that particular migraine attack disappeared, and now I am astounded that I have not had an attack to equal the severity or the frequency of them since.

'As any migraine sufferer can imagine, I am very thankful that I tried cranial osteopathy as there are numerous benefits: I only need a reduced dosage of medication now to control the migraine (instead of it controlling my life!); I can again look forward to holidays; I am able to work to my full capacity; I am now able to study for a law degree. None of these would have been possible to consider, let alone endeavour, without the help and treatment of cranial osteopathy.'

Bren Taylor

Crystal Therapy

Origins

Crystals and precious gems abound in myths and legends, and have been regarded as possessing mystical and healing powers for centuries. Their rarity, clarity and beauty have long been associated with enlightenment and power, and, in fact, it was this traditional belief in the special properties of crystals that gave rise to the more recent phenomenon of crystal-ball gazing. Crystal therapists maintain that crystals are 'ice from heaven', a form of ancient energy and solidified light, and are capable of transmitting their own energies to the human body to promote well-being and healing.

What is crystal therapy?

Crystal or gemstone therapy is designed to promote physical, psychological and spiritual well-being. Crystals themselves may be multifaceted, cubic or prism-shaped; it is the perfection of the atomic structure, the shape and the clarity of the crystal that are thought to help patients approach perfection themselves. Practitioners claim that not only can people get better, but that the healing forces of crystals can also help sick animals and improve the overall aura of buildings and the environment generally. There are literally thousands of minerals which may exist in crystal form, and these may be used by people who practise purely as crystal therapists, or by other complementary therapists, such as aromatherapists, kinesiologists, movement therapists and spiritual healers, who use crystals as part of their healing repertoire.

How does it work?

Crystal therapists claim that crystals and gemstones give off electromagnetic energy which can transmit healing forces to the energy circulating along meridians within the human body. They believe that many kinds of rock, precious or otherwise, have a consciousness which can communicate with our soul or spirit. Quartz, for example, is capable of generating enough piezo-electricity to power watches and other small computers. In a similar way, other crystals can radiate energy and have a beneficial effect on the body. Amber is claimed to have a calming effect which will help treat or prevent depression, and moonstone is thought to control hormonal and emotional imbalances. Some therapists place crystals or stones in purified water and expose them to the sun's rays in order to transfer the energy from the crystals into the water. Others use a pendulum or pyramid to tap into the crystal's energy. Sitting under a pyramid or placing drops of the energized water under the tongue are therefore common methods of treatment, although merely having crystals placed at certain points around the body is the most usual method.

Is crystal therapy effective?

Crystal therapy is not usually used to remedy precise medical conditions, and therefore no scientific trials have been conducted on its efficacy. This therapy is used holistically to improve a patient's spiritual well-being, and to make them feel better generally. Anecdotal reports suggest that it is particularly helpful in abolishing symptoms of stress and the discomfort of low back pain and rheumatic ailments.

What form might the treatment take?

There is nothing to stop somebody going out and purchasing crystals themselves, but many prefer to see a qualified crystal healer first. The therapist will generally enquire about the patient's lifestyle, symptoms and general outlook, and might ask the patient to sit in a chair, or lie flat on the floor or on a couch. There is no need to remove any clothing. Since there is no standard routine for this kind of consultation, what the therapist does next will vary, but he or she may place crystals around you, may give you a crystal to hold, or may place them on any of the body's energy centres, commonly known as chakras. Sometimes the therapist holds the crystals. His or her aim is to direct the ancient healing energy into the patient, thereby enabling the patient to heal themselves, using the crystal merely as a catalyst. The choice of any crystals used will depend entirely on what the therapist considers is correct for the patient and their condition. He or she might place the crystal over the location of any discomfort, and might, for example, place garnet on the forehead chakra if the patient is depressed. In addition, before the end of the consultation, the therapist will provide the patient with crystals to take home, together with advice about how to preserve their properties. The patient will be encouraged to 'dedicate' the crystal by saying out loud that it will be used to help and heal, and not for any untoward or evil purposes.

What problems are helped by crystal therapy

Gemstone and crystal therapy is really designed to be used holistically to reduce stress, to improve well-being and to raise consciousness and awareness. It is said to help the body heal itself by sorting out its own energy imbalances, and it claims to improve conditions as far-ranging as arthritis and back pain right through to depression, palpitations and fatigue.

Is it safe?

Since these ancient stones contain primeval energy that is capable of causing harm as well as healing, therapists often recommend that a patient dedicates their crystal to be used only for the power of good. Theoretically, no harm can be done using crystal therapy unless, of course, serious conditions are ignored or the patient is discouraged from seeking a proper diagnosis and treatment at the same time as exploring this particular type of therapy. Since the healing is subtle and non-invasive, there would appear to be no condition and no age for which this therapy is contra-indicated.

How can I find a crystal therapist?

Anybody can set themselves up as a crystal therapist, and clearly there is much scope for abuse. Just as in other unregulated complementary therapies, clients should be extremely careful about revealing anything of their medical history or lifestyle to unfamiliar people who could use the information for their own benefit. However, the Affiliation of Crystal Healing Organizations (ACHO) was established in 1988 and is an umbrella organization ensuring that all registered therapists have undergone a minimum of two years part-time training, are indemnified against malpractice and also abide by a recognized code of conduct.

How much will it cost?

Usually sessions will be priced at about £20, although many

practitioners may make special provisions for unemployed or elderly patients. The precious gemstones embedded in the crown jewels are valued at hundreds of thousands of pounds, but interested parties will be relieved to hear that crystals with healing properties are obtainable for as little as 10p or so. Whether the value of the stone confers extra healing energy is surprisingly rarely discussed.

The sceptic's view

Crystal therapy is yet more arrant nonsense perpetrated by people who believe in some mysterious ancient power that can influence our mind, body and soul. That patently unqualified and untrained people can facilitate the transmission of such non-existent power reinforces its nonsensical basis, and the sceptic would sincerely advise any vulnerable person with problems to stay well clear of such blatant quackery. By all means use a quartz power source in your wrist-watch, but do not go to the bother of placing them neatly around your bed in the hope of warding off evil spirits. As for the higher consciousness which is supposed to exist in all solid matter, any one who believes this can only be one step short of taking their rock for a therapeutic walk, as they do in the mad environs of Los Angeles and its suburbs.

The therapist's view

The crystal therapist recognizes that the malaise, lassitude and general sense of being run down which pervades modern society, is spectacularly not improved by conventional treatments. There is a polarity and dilution of soul and spirit which is partly to blame. The holistic and subtle treatment that is crystal therapy enables the patient to tune into the ancient power of gemstone in order to restore some spiritual well-being, and often this can lead to significant improvement in the patient's health and general outlook. The precious stones were formed hundreds of thousands of years ago and have withstood holocausts and natural disasters time after time. The energy and vitality which has enabled them to do so can also facilitate natural healing powers in the body. It is a safe and inexpensive method of treatment which allows everybody the importance of hope.

The patient's view

'Nothing, but nothing, seemed to alleviate my chronic fatigue and exhaustion. First they thought it was the menopause, then an underactive thyroid, and then, when all that had been excluded by medical tests, they said I was bored or depressed. I told them I was neither of these, and that I simply wanted to have more energy and get-up-and-go. I went to a health exhibition and was intrigued by a stand devoted to crystal therapy. For a laugh, I had a treatment there and then, and was amazed to discover how brilliant I felt on the way home, and all the following week. I ended up purchasing a selection of crystals which I place under my pillow and scatter around my living-room and on my desk at work, and I have never looked back. Lots of people think I have become a bit wacky, but what the hell – it works.'

Barbara Nagle

Herbal Medicine

(see also Chinese Herbal Medicine)

Origins

The use of herbs as medicine has been known to all cultures for thousands of years, and must be one of the oldest therapies of all. Not only has herbalism been popular in the West, but has also formed an integral part of ancient Chinese medicine and of African and Indian therapies since the beginning of time. In European countries, herbal remedies are currently enjoying a resurgence of popularity following a temporary eclipse during the 1950s and 1960s, when more powerful pharmaceutical drugs were enjoying a honeymoon period. Today, some 5 million people in Britain regularly buy herbal treatments, spending nearly £30 million each year. There are many perceived attractions to herbal medicines: their relative cheapness; they are derived from natural products; they are free of synthetic materials, such as preservatives and additives; compared to many more powerful pharmaceutical medications, they are gentle, and less likely to produce side effects.

What is herbal medicine?

It is a treatment that exploits the healing qualities of plants, herbs, flowers and trees to support our own innate healing systems in overcoming environmental insults and challenges. Herbalists maintain that when our own vital life-force is run down by stress, pollution and bad diet, we become ill, and that our symptoms of ill-health represent the consequences of our own body's healing mechanisms trying to maintain harmonious balance within the body. Just as orthodox doctors see a raised temperature as the result of our body's fight against an invading micro-organism, herbalists see a patient's symptoms as a sign that their body is attempting to overcome the underlying condition itself. However, herbalists go on to say that as well as fighting disease, herbs are capable of preventing disease from happening in the first place, whilst supporting the immune system, detoxifying the body and promoting long-term good health.

Herbal medicine has been administered throughout history, by Cleopatra's beauticians and by the medical establishment patronized by Henry VIII, but in modern times the traditional applications of herbal extracts have been updated and refined to take into account state-of-the-art scientific research. Information originally contained in Nicholas Culpeper's early work on herbalism, *English Physician and Complete Herbal*, first published in 1653, has been developed and matured and has now found favour with well-respected bodies such as the World Health Organization, who have long regarded the benefits of herbal medicine sympathetically and enthusiastically.

How does it work?

Herbal preparations derived from flowers, roots, barks, seeds and nuts consist of a number of different chemical components that are known to have curative properties in humans. One of the better-known examples is acetyl salicylic acid, or aspirin, which was originally found in willow bark. Another is digitalis, which occurs naturally in foxglove. During the early part of the twentieth century, the majority of drugs used by conventional doctors were in fact extracted from herbs and many still are.

What is becoming increasingly clear, however, is that although the active ingredients can be taken individually from plants and synthesized in the laboratory, the herbs often work best in their natural whole state as the other chemical components in the whole plant seem to work synergistically, enhancing the beneficial effects whilst avoiding any side effects. One example of this synergism is the effect garlic produces when used as an antibiotic. Synthetic antibiotics, like penicillin, are widely known to produce side effects, such as diarrhoea, because they kill the useful bacteria in the large intestine that are needed for normal digestion at the same time as killing the harmful bacteria that are causing the infection, be it pneumonia, meningitis or a skin abscess. Garlic, on the other hand, works as a natural antibiotic without causing harm to the normal gut flora, nor making yeast infection more likely as a consequence of it being taken.

Herbalists are trained to recommend specific herbs for the individual patient rather than prescribing set formulas for specific illnesses or symptoms. For example. a patient suffering from insomnia and irritable bowel syndrome (IBS) might be prescribed Valerian for the insomnia rather than Jamaican dogweed or Passion flower (both of which have similar properties to Valerian), because Valerian has an additional calming effect on the digestive system and would therefore be helpful for somebody suffering from both insomnia and IBS. In addition, many medical herbalists believe that because certain herbs contain a variety of active compounds naturally blended together, they are 'adaptogenic' and may help disorders that are resistant to orthodox treatment. Ginseng, for example, is considered adaptogenic because it has different effects in different people balancing energy levels by reducing energy where it is overactive and increasing it where it is depressed. Camomile is thought to have similar regulatory and adaptogenic powers in the intestine. This is why herbalists are so enthusiastic about these natural products; they consider they are capable of achieving things which synthetically manufactured pharmaceutical medications singly cannot.

The remedies themselves come in many shapes and forms. They can be taken orally or rubbed on the skin, and they come as tinctures, decoctions, infusions, tablets, capsules, compresses, poultices and herbal baths. Each is made up differently.

Tinctures

These are produced by soaking the useful part of the herb in alcohol to preserve it. Tinctures are the most common formulation taken internally. Only small quantities are taken and the tinctures keep for long periods of time.

Decoctions

These use the bark, roots, nuts and seeds of herbs in either fresh or dried form. They are made into a decoction by putting one teaspoon of the herb material into one cup of boiling water, and then simmering for about 10 minutes. The liquid is then strained and the decoction drunk hot.

Infusions

Like decoctions these are less concentrated than tinctures. They are made up in the same way as decoctions but using the flowers, stems or leaves of the herbs. Infusions may be made more palatable by sweetening them with honey, if required. Certain herbs, like comfrey, are denatured by boiling, so these are best infused in cold water for anything up to a day.

Capsules and tablets

Just like over-the-counter medicines from the chemist or doctor, these are more convenient for those in a hurry or for those who are put off by the taste of other oral preparations. To make them, extracts of herbs are compounded into a pill or capsule with chalk or gelatine.

Herbal creams

Used to accelerate healing of sprains and bruises, these are rubbed into the skin in the normal way. Preparations are also available to moisturize dry, flakey skin, and I know of many a television make-up artist who would use nothing else for facial blemishes.

Poultices

These are made from herbs which are crushed and mixed into a paste with warm water. Like orthodox medical poultices they are applied on some form of dressing to boils, spots or inflamed joints in an attempt to draw out the inflammation and infection.

Compresses

These may be hot or cold, and involve soaking a medical dressing in a herbal infusion, and then applying it to a painful or inflamed area. Generally speaking, hot compresses are used for stiff, cool joints, and cold compresses are used for red, inflamed, swollen joints.

Herbal baths

Many people enjoy a scented bath without ever imagining they have made use of herbal medicine. However, the fragrances used in many commercial products will include the same herbal aromas (even if synthetic) that are used in traditional herbalism. Lavender, pine, lemon balm and elderflower are all popular. Alternatively, the herbs can be purchased in a muslin bag which is then hung from the bath taps allowing hot water to run through it. Aromatherapists use essential oils in a similar way, but apply it to the bath water itself (see page 118). The theory is that the pores of the skin absorb some of the helpful properties, while others are inhaled into the respiratory system where they pass into the bloodstream.

Commonly used herbs and their beneficial properties include the following:

- *Aloe vera*, used in gel or oral form, is said to be good for minor burns, scalds or sunburn, and is used by some babywipe manufacturers as a preventative of nappy rash and ammoniacal dermatitis.
- *Calendula*, in cream form, may be applied to small wounds, abrasions and areas of skin inflammation.
- *Echinacea* is very popular now for the treatment of colds, coughs, sore throats and influenza.
- *Evening primrose* oil has a wide following amongst sufferers of premenstrual syndrome and of eczema, but it is also useful to counteract the unpleasant symptoms of the menopause and works as a hangover cure.
- *Garlic* is very commonly used now to reduce cholesterol levels in the blood and to prevent respiratory infections. It is known to have antiseptic and antifungal actions and is also used for bronchitis and thrush infections.
- *Ginger* is one of the few perfectly safe remedies a pregnant woman can take for the common symptom of indigestion, so it is used to treat morning sickness as well as travel sickness, wind, arthritis and circulation problems. The natural root can be chewed, or ginger can be taken in capsule form or as an infusion. Orthodox doctors even take it with their whisky at night in the form of a Whisky Mac.
- *Ginkgo biloba* comes from the leaves of the maidenhair tree and is thought to mop up free radicals in the body, thereby acting as an antioxidant (see page 257). It is also said to boost circulation, to help thin the blood and to treat tinnitus (an inconvenient and sometimes distressing buzzing or ringing noise in the ear).
- *Ginseng* is used to stimulate the immune system and activity of the brain. Used for thousands of years by the Chinese, it has a number of other applications including boosting a flagging sex drive.
- *Lavender* is used to alleviate stress and tension, to bring about relaxation, and to cure insomnia.
- *Meadowsweet* as an infusion has a mild analgesic effect and can be useful in treating heart burn.

- *Mistletoe*, now marketed as *iskador*, has been used to treat cancer, although its efficacy in this area has been challenged by the conventional medical fraternity.
- *Peppermint* is used for irritable bowel syndrome, flatulence and wind, heartburn, indigestion, headaches and colds.
- *St John's wort*, used for depression, has been the subject of several clinical trials, the results of which provide fairly compelling evidence that it has a significant beneficial effect.
- *Tea tree oil* has marked antifungal and antiseptic properties and may be used for stings, abrasions and cuts as well as on warts and cold sores.

Is herbal medicine effective?

Several randomized controlled studies have shown St John's wort (Hypericum) to be effective in the treatment of clinical depression. In 1996 meta-analysis, which is the combined analysis of a number of completely separate major clinical trials, confirmed that St John's wort was more effective than placebo treatment and was a good, safe, mild antidepressant. Other work has shown that echinacea purpurea seems to be able to stimulate the immune system, to protect people against simple colds and coughs, and to accelerate recovery from them once they have become established. Even in the days before penicillin in the 1940s, conventional doctors were using echinacea to treat even serious conditions such as meningitis, diphtheria and tuberculosis. More than a thousand studies have been conducted on the benefits of garlic, and there is now a broad consensus of opinion that it is useful for circulatory problems as well as helping to prevent respiratory infection. Other work has strongly suggested that Valerian has a significant action in the treatment of insomnia, and that oil of evening primrose can reduce the symptoms of premenstrual syndrome.

There are, of course, hundreds of different herbs whose characteristics are exploited by commercial organizations making a variety of health claims about their properties. Some of these products contain very small amounts of the original herb, and some of this may not appear in any active and biologically useful form. Furthermore, many of the health-giving claims that are made have never been substantiated by any scientific study.

What form might the treatment take?

Although it is possible to buy an over-the-counter herbal remedy, this goes against the grain, to some extent, because herbal therapists believe that treatments should be tailored to the individual and should not be dispensed empirically with a particular illness in mind. Many people require guidance, at least to begin with, in selecting the correct treatment, and are therefore happy to book an appointment with a trained herbalist.

The first consultation is likely to last about one hour, where a holistic approach will be taken to assessing the patient's condition. Herbalists themselves are not allowed by law to recommend a treatment to a patient they have not seen in person. An enquiry will be made into the patient's medical history, lifestyle, relationships, work, diet, emotional state and personality. The patient will be asked if they are currently taking any medication. In fact, 'medical' herbalists have also been trained along conventional lines, having studied anatomy, physiology and biochemistry, and the patient is usually physically examined in much the same way as they would be at any NHS surgery.

Once the diagnosis has been reached, the herbalist will prescribe a herbal remedy in one of the forms described above. However, the therapist will not choose the treatment in order to remedy a specific condition, such as arthritis or depression, but will select it on the basis that it is designed to help the body's own healing system to overcome the underlying condition that is caused the symptoms. For those people having trouble sleeping, for example, a remedy to alleviate the stress that is causing the problem might be selected, and for someone suffering from anxiety, a treatment designed to have a calming effect on an over-stimulated nervous system might be chosen. Most herbalists would expect to see improvement in a patient's condition within

2–3 months at the most, and even the most enthusiastic patients are not usually seen any more regularly than about once every three weeks.

What problems are helped by herbal medicine?

Although almost any medical ailment can lend itself to herbal treatment, certain problems seem to respond better than others. Non-specific ailments, such as irritable bowel syndrome, ME (myalgic encephalomyelitis), eczema and other dry skin problems like psoriasis, urinary problems and indigestion, all seem to respond well. Some people even keep a herbal first-aid kit in their homes to treat commonly arising situations like scalds, cuts, abrasions and sprains as herbal creams, ointments, poultices and tablets have a wide range of applications. Good herbalists, however, are aware that herbal medicine has its limitations and will never pretend that it can deal with serious and life-threatening conditions such as AIDS, diabetes and cancer. Presented with these problems, herbalists are very conscientious about advising patients to consult more appropriate therapists.

Is it safe?

Although herbal medicines, by and large, have a better safety record than pharmaceutical preparations, they, too, are capable of causing side effects. The fact that they are natural does not make them harmless. Penny royal and broom, for example, can cause miscarriages, and feverfew, often used to treat migraine, can bring on mouth ulcers. Ragwort and bear-berry have been associated with liver damage, and comfrey preparations were taken off the market in the UK because they, too, can cause liver damage as they contain pyrrolizidine alkaloids. The Poisons Unit at Guy's and St Thomas's Hospital kept records on the side effects of herbal medicines over five years and published a report in 1996 which found likely links between adverse symptoms and herbal products in over 600 cases. It is also worth bearing in mind that some herbal preparations can interfere with drugs prescribed by orthodox doctors. Vitamin K, for example, can interact with anticoagulants taken by people with valvular disease of the heart or people who have had blood clots in the lungs or legs. Kelp can interact with antithyroid drugs, and ginseng can interfere with the normal action of an antidepressant called phenelzine. To complicate matters, many herbal remedies contain several active ingredients working synergistically, some of which have never been properly identified.

Excessive intake of certain herbs can be toxic and as the quality control of certain oriental herbs is poor, it is also possible that contamination with potentially harmful substances may occur. Luckily, quality control on most Western herbs is much tighter, but even then, some potentially harmful products can slip through the net, often in the form of bulk imports or mail order products. It was proposed as recently as 1994 that the agency which regulates medicinal products for human use in Britain, the Medicines Control Agency (MCA) should license all herbal medicines, but in view of the unprecedented number of people who objected to these proposals the plan was dropped. The pressure from a market turning over nearly £30 million a year from the sale of herbs was too much to resist, and the 5 million people who regularly buy these products see that licensing would raise prices. The MCA now only licenses a very few herbal remedies which are classed as medicines, and these few have to be tested by law. Eighty per cent of herbal remedies remain unlicensed.

Since we know herbs have the potential to cause harm, who is therefore responsible for their prescription? The Medicines Act of 1968 does not demand that a herbalist supplying herbal products to a patient has a licence, nor does the practitioner need to supply any list of ingredients. The application of the herbalist's prescription and its safety remain his or her own clinical responsibility. However, it is the manufacturer rather than the herbalist who is responsible if the herbalist merely dispenses treatment produced by someone else. It is good advice, therefore, to restrict the purchase of herbal remedies to the home market, not to buy by mail order, to buy only products which list their ingredients and not to rely on herbal treatments for serious diseases. The dose should never be exceeded, treatment should not be taken for a prolonged length of time, and any side effects should be reported immediately. Only experienced people should pick herbs growing wild and it is always a good idea to ask your GP about any pre-existing conditions if you are considering taking any herbal remedy.

How can I find a herbalist?

Herbalism is unlicensed, and anyone can set themselves up as a herbalist. Look, therefore, for a herbalist who is a member of the National Institute of Medical Herbalists and who has the initials MNIH (Member of the National Institute of Medical Herbalists) after their name. They abide by a code of practice and ethics, and have a professional indemnity to protect themselves as well as their patients in case of problems. All members have undergone lengthy degree courses in herbal medicine, which incorporate much of the ground covered by conventional doctors in their training. There are courses available for qualified GPs and others, which are less lengthy. It is hoped in the future that a single supervisory body will one day be set up to encompass both western and oriental herbal medicine under one regulatory umbrella.

How much will it cost?

Consultations will normally cost in the region of £25, with a further £10–15 spent on prescribed preparations. A very few NHS GPs are herbalists in their own right, but for the majority of people, it is highly unlikely that you can obtain free herbal treatment.

The sceptic's view

The ill sceptic wants something that will work effectively and fast. He or she doesn't want to be seen rooting about in the garden for greenery that is difficult to identify, and which has to be boiled up before it can be taken in the hope that it will relieve symptoms. This is for the birds. Why have a multi-million-pound pharmaceutical industry which can identify and concentrate the active ingredients in these plants, and make them into a convenient and pleasantly flavoured tablet in a matter of hours without you even having to get your hands dirty? At least the pharmaceutical company has taken the trouble to keep the preparations relatively safe, and they have to, otherwise the sceptics would sue them. Herbal preparations, on the other hand, are just as expensive as prescription drugs, and are also capable of producing toxic effects. It is an unlicensed industry which freely admits it can do little to treat serious illness, and merely panders to the superstitious folklore of ignorant people from days gone by. The idea of an 'adaptogenic' herb like peppermint adapting its action in order to remedy a troubled digestive system, caused by any number of different conditions, is too crass to be credible. No, give the sceptic a powerful but effective drug any day rather than a gentle but ineffective herb.

The therapist's view

'It is a joy to work with the healing properties of flowers, plants, trees and herbs, to stimulate the body's natural healing powers. Herbalism is such a gentle yet natural form of treatment, with its safety and efficacy steeped in centuries of experience. The treatments are versatile, coming in so many various forms that there is always something to suit every individual with their specific problems. I find it particularly useful for skin conditions, such as psoriasis and eczema, and I have had particular success treating cystitis and disorders relating to the digestive system. I treat the elderly, the very young, and women who are expecting, and I encourage all my clients to build up a herbal first-aid kit to have in the home as well.'

Mary Timms

The patient's view

'I have always been convinced about the healing power of herbs ever since

my mother used remedies which have been traditionally passed down through families for generations. I used ginger successfully for getting rid of morning sickness when I was expecting my children, and I have used ginseng at times when I have felt worn out and totally lacking in energy. I swear by echinacea and garlic to ward of colds and coughs, and now that I have begun to make my own concoctions and infusions, have never felt so well in myself and gone so long without medical problems. My husband's depression was vastly improved by St John's wort and I even got rid of my son's nits with tea tree oil. I have seen so many side effects from powerful pharmaceutical drugs, and I wonder whether we really need to use these so frequently when nature has provided us with such a wonderful assortment of healing herbs already.'

Gemma Bridges

Homeopathy

Origins

Homeopathic principles originate as far back as the fifth century BC, when the father of medicine, Hippocrates, attempted to distinguish between disease itself and how it affected our individual bodies. He believed that symptoms were merely manifestations of a reaction inside people to ill-health, and that each person might react differently to the same disorder.

The importance of the unique individual remains a central cornerstone in modern homeopathy, but it was the German physician and chemist Samuel Hahnemann (1755–1843) who resurrected the principles of homeopathy and popularized them in the modern world. Although Hahnemann was trained in conventional medicine, he became disillusioned by many of the barbaric surgical procedures and practices of the day, and by the powerful medications that were used without any sound rational basis, and which caused such appalling side effects. Casting aside his successful practice in Saxony, he became a translator and in that occupational capacity came across a work entitled *A Treatise on Materia Medica* written by the Scottish physician Dr William Cullen. Cullen stated in his book that quinine was an effective remedy for malaria, and Hahnemann wanted to discover why this should be so. Experimenting on himself, he took quinine and found that over a period of time he developed many of the symptoms of malaria, despite being free of the disease itself. Excited by his research, he conducted further investigations which he termed 'provings'. He gave a variety of compounds of animal, mineral and vegetable origin to a number of willing volunteers, then observed them for any resulting symptoms. The symptoms which occurred most commonly were called 'first line' symptoms, less common symptoms were called 'second line' symptoms and those that occurred only rarely were called 'third line' symptoms. Eventually, Hahnemann was able to develop a drug picture for each of the substances he investigated. His next step was to draw a symptoms picture for every patient he saw, before administering any treatment. The end result of his work was a publication called *The Law of Similars*, which was printed in 1796.

Hahnemann also proposed three essential principles which were to form the basis of modern homeopathy. Firstly, he stated that if large doses of a substance promoted symptoms in a healthy person, then much smaller doses of the same substance could cure people who already had similar symptoms of disease. Hahnemann thought this was because nature did not allow people to suffer from two similar diseases at any one time. The second principle was the 'minimum dose principle' which stated that the greater the dilution of a curative substance, the more potent and effective it became. This was known as 'potentization'. The third main principle was that of 'whole person prescribing'. When treating any individual, the homeopath takes into account the patient's personality, mood and temperament as well as their physical and emotional health before any remedy is dispensed. On this basis, two patients with exactly the same symptoms might well be treated with entirely different medication. This is of course in great contrast to the situation in conventional medical circles.

What is homeopathy?

Basically, homeopathy is a holistic therapy that uses preparations of animal, vegetable and mineral origin in a variety of dilutions to cure a person's illness. Its principles are basically to treat 'like with like' and to use remedies that stimulate the body to heal itself. The name homeopathy is, in fact, derived from two Greek words, *homios* meaning like and *pathos* meaning suffering. Although the Chinese call the energy within each person 'Chi', and the Indians call it 'Prana', Hahnemann referred to the internal healing power within us as the 'vital force'. He believed that his homeopathic remedies rallied and organized the vital force, enabling it to recover from illness and to restore the organism to perfect health. In contrast to orthodox medicine, which prescribes medicines like antidotes to abolish symptoms, homeopathy takes a substance which would cause symptoms in a healthy person, and uses it to cure identical symptoms in a person who has a disease. By way of example, a conventional doctor would prescribe an anti-nausea medication for sickness, whereas a homeopathic physician might prescribe nux vomica which in high doses would cause the very symptoms it was designed to remedy. Homeopathic remedies, however are only given in minute amounts, the dilution of the substance prescribed being so weak that little or none of the original substance within it could ever be detected by laboratory means.

Homeopathic solutions and treatments are prepared by taking the original substance, be it plant, mineral or animal, and producing a solution from it known as the 'mother tincture'. This is then diluted several times. Each time dilution takes place, the liquid is shaken vigorously, a process known as 'succussion'. Remember that the more dilute the solution becomes, the more effective homeopaths believe it to be. Dilutions may be decimal or centesimal. The decimal gradation is tenfold so a 1x solution is a 1 in 10 dilution of the mother tincture, and a 2x solution is a 1 in 100 dilution, and so on. In the centesimal scale, the dilutions occur in hundreds. A 1c solution is a 1 in 100 dilution, and a 2c solution, a 1 in 10, 000 dilution, and so on. For minor symptoms, such as headaches, aches and pains, and fatigue, a 6 potency or a 6c dilution is generally employed.

How does it work?

Homeopathy is supposed to work by boosting the innate healing power within the body. It sees symptoms not as a result of illness itself, but as a manifestation of the body's struggle to heal itself. Homeopaths believe that the remedies contain a vibrational energy which provides the information required to enable the body to overcome whatever disorder is affecting it. Homeopathic remedies have been likened to a computer disc, which incorporates vast amounts of data, but which when analysed would merely reveal a piece of plastic and traces of other synthetic substances. Similarly, analysis of a homeopathic medicine might show merely water and the diluting media ethanol and lactose, but it could not hope to show the information within. The principle of homeopathy has also been likened to the principle of vaccination, whereby a tiny amount of a substance is injected into the body to promote an overwhelming recruitment of the immune system, so that when the body is confronted with a virulent and potentially harmful virus, such as smallpox or measles, good health can be maintained. This analogy is not quite accurate, however, as in any vaccination there is a recognizable micro-organism, albeit in altered form, which can be chemically identified, whereas in homeopathic remedies, especially in the higher dilutions, there is nothing whatsoever to see or find.

Is homeopathy effective?

In the 1850s, in the early days of homeopathy, patients actually fared better when they were treated in a homeopathic hospital than they did in conventional hospitals, and this did much to help promote its acceptance. Apparently, the death rate was 40 per cent better when homeopathic remedies were used. Since then, there have been many attempts to prove scientifically the efficacy of homeopathy, although most scientists would probably agree that the jury is still out on the interpretation of the findings. In 1991 the *British Medical Journal* reviewed over 100 clinically controlled trials, concluding that 75 per cent of them showed encouraging findings. Another study set up at Glasgow's Royal Infirmary showed that homeopathic remedies worked better than a placebo in patients with asthma who were allergic to the house dust mite. Other trials have shown that patients with chronic skin complaints and migraine also fared better than patients taking just a placebo, which is interesting because sceptics have always argued that the benefits of homeopathy are merely no more than than a placebo itself. Unfortunately, few of these trials have compared the effects of homeopathic remedies to those of conventional remedies, but this in itself is extremely difficult to do in a controlled clinical trial because, since the very basis of homeopathy means that patients are treated as individuals rather than groups of people with similar symptoms, it is difficult to find two large identical groups of patients on whom to carry out the trial. Perhaps the popularity of homeopathy speaks for itself. It is the third most commonly used complementary therapy, and demand for its remedies is continually growing, with the five NHS homeopathic hospitals seeing more patients year after year, than ever before. Furthermore there are now many conventionally trained doctors who are using homeopathy in addition to their conventional medicines and treatments, and this is a phenomenon which is likely to develop further.

What form might the treatment take?

Since one of the essential tenets of homeopathic treatment is to tailor the specific remedy to the individual, the best way to seek treatment is to consult a qualified homeopath. However, a number of remedies, which have been prepared to treat a variety of common symptoms, can be bought off the shelf from pharmacies and health food shops, and can be taken satisfactorily on a do-it-yourself basis at home. By and large, acute symptoms require a 6c dilution, and less acute ailments are usually treated with a 30c potency solution. It might be recommended that the treatment should be taken every 2 hours for the first six doses, followed up by, say, 3-times-a-day dosage between meals. Treatment may come in the form of pills, granules, liquids or powders, and they come in two types, the classical or single-remedy products, and the combined remedies which are combinations of several single remedies and which are generally thought to be best at treating disorders diagnosed by conventional means. Rhus tox 6c, for example, is recommended for nappy rash, stiff and painful muscles, rheumatic type pains and itching blisters, and Cantharis 6c is prescribed to treat cystitis, blisters, scalds, burns and stinging or burning of the skin. The problem with DIY homeopathy is that the remedies are not selected for the patient as an individual, and consumers often do not have enough expertise to make the right choice.

When a qualified homeopath is consulted, he or she would initially enquire about the patient as a person, and about their personality, outlook and emotional and physical health. As they are taking the patient's case history, they would ask about any previous medical history, and inquire into the medical history of the patient's family. Questions would also be asked about the patient's social life, nutritional status, place of work, how the person feels and about any particular likes and dislikes. Once the detailed consultation is complete, the homeopath will choose a remedy according to what they have been told and whatever is most likely to solve the problem. The homeopath would also probably explain the rule of 12 to the patient. This means that the speed at which the symptoms respond to treatment will depend on the length of time the symptoms have already been present. For example, if the patient has been unwell for a year, it would take one twelfth of that time, i. e. one month, before any improvement would expect to be noticed. He or she will also explain that there might initially be an exacerbation of the symptoms, called an 'aggravation reaction', which the homeopath regards as a positive indication that treatment is beginning to work and has begun to eradicate those manifestations of the disorder which have been underlying the patient's symptoms all along. Patients should be reassured that aggravation reactions are usually short-lived and are certainly not severe. Treatment may only require a first or second visit to the homeopath, but clearly the duration of treatment depends on the nature and severity of the original illness.

What problems are helped by homeopathy?

Common and irritating symptoms such as nausea and vomiting, diarrhoea, constipation, colds and coughs, and allergies seem to respond best, but more significant and chronic conditions, such as arthritis and fibrositis and skin conditions such as psoriasis and eczema, may improve too. Irritable bowel syndrome, migraine and other headaches, premenstrual tension and any stress-related, emotional and mental disorders have all been helped in individual patients by this form of complementary therapy.

Is it safe?

One of the beauties of homeopathic remedies, which has endeared it to so many people in this day and age of drug and medicine awareness, is that the remedies are completely safe for everyone. They can therefore be taken by pregnant women and the elderly, and even babies. Since lactose is the basic substrate for the pills, the only effect a baby taking an accidental overdose of homeopathic medicines would suffer is looser stools. Homeopathic remedies are often administered to animals and no side effects have been noted in these situations either. The only real danger in homeopathy lies in seeing an unqualified and unregistered practitioner who is unable to spot serious disease, and where the patient is prescribed a remedy at the expense of a significant problem being neglected or ignored. The best policy is to make sure you see a conventional doctor at the same time.

How can I find a homeopath?

There are two types of homeopath, those who have orthodox qualifications and additional training in homeopathy, and those who are trained in homeopathy alone and who do not have any orthodox medical qualifications. In fact, homeopathy is unique in complementary medicine in that there is a Faculty of Homeopathy established by an Act of Parliament, which oversees the training and registration of homeopathic practitioners. There are five NHS homeopathic hospitals in Britain, and there are some 300 or so medically qualified doctors who are registered as homeopaths, and are entitled to place the letters MFHom after their names. There are also a few GPs who have not undergone the six-month post-graduate course at the Faculty, but who still prescribe homeopathic medicine to their patients. The other professional homeopaths, who are not qualified as doctors, can nevertheless join the Society of Homeopaths and place RSHom after their names, or FSHom once they become fellows, having undergone a recognized course at an approved college. It is important to realize, too, that anybody can legitimately call themselves a homeopath without any qualification whatsoever, as the discipline is as yet unregulated. The NHS homeopathic hospitals are found in London, Glasgow, Bristol, Liverpool and Tunbridge Wells.

How much will it cost?

Although costs vary, the first consultation will be in the region of £60–70, with follow-up appointments being cheaper. NHS GPs can refer you to an NHS homeopathic hospital provided they are fund-holders, and even if they are not, your doctor may be able to arrange with the local health authority for you to have homeopathic treatment. It is an interesting sign of the times that many private health insurance companies now allow cover for this kind of therapy.

The sceptic's view

The sceptic would agree that homeopathy is based on a wonderfully imaginative idea, but would have to raise an eyebrow over the principle of potentization, because in the dilutions used in the treatment, there is often no traceable element of the original substance to be found. The philosophy that weaker is more effective is totally alien to the sceptic's way of thinking, and the disbeliever will also attribute much of the anecdotal success of homeopathy to the placebo effect. Grudgingly, he or she might have to accept that demand for homeopathic remedies is increasing dramatically, and that many members of the established orthodox medical profession are becoming increasingly seduced by their charms. However, whilst the practice remains unregulated, and whilst there are totally unqualified people out there pushing unproven homeopathic treatments, the public is still potentially vulnerable. The sceptic would concede, however, that, like Hahnemann, the originator of homeopathic medicine who did not like the brutality of contemporary medical practice, many modern doctors who have had enough of the blood and guts philosophy associated with many of the invasive techniques used in modern medicine, would find much within the gentle and safe practice of homeopathy to commend it.

The therapist's view

'Homeopathy is a dynamic system of healing that attempts to improve overall experience of health on mental, emotional and physical levels. One of the most exciting aspects of this therapy is the way in which each patient is viewed as an individual who experiences ill-health in their own unique way. As a result, the homeopathic remedy that is selected must fit the symptoms experienced as closely as possible for improvement to take place. This is why homeopathy is sometimes referred to as a 'patient-centred' form of therapy, since it focuses on bringing the whole person into balance, rather than providing medicines that temporarily relieve symptoms.

'This extremely human aspect of homeopathic treatment was brought home to me in a personal way when my husband consulted a homeopathic practitioner sixteen years ago. At that time I knew very little about homeopathic theory, and had few preconceptions about what his treatment might involve. As I learned more about homeopathy in practice, I was astonished and fascinated with what I perceived to be an unusually flexible and human approach to medical care.

'The attention paid to exploring the links between physical, mental and emotional problems appealed strongly to me, as well as the amount of advice that was given about general improvements in lifestyle that would be supportive of an improvement in overall well-being.

'In addition, I was delighted to discover that the homeopathic perspective, in common with other holistic systems of healing, such as traditional Chinese medicine and Western medical herbalism, involves a very positive approach to the treatment of illness. Homeopathic medicine has more to do with health promotion than disease management. As a result, strong emphasis is put on the need to strengthen the body's own capacity to fight illness through appropriate homeopathic prescribing.

'Finally, perhaps the most exciting aspect of homeopathic treatment is the way that it can be used to relieve a broad spectrum of conditions and problems. Homeopaths are regularly called on to treat a broad range of problems in babies and children, while the elderly can benefit greatly from homeopathic help. In addition, homeopathic treatment is a popular option for dealing with chronic conditions such as eczema, asthma, hay fever, migraine, arthritis, digestive problems, premenstrual syndrome, and recurrent infections. Those who suffer from stress-related emotional problems, such as anxiety and depression, can also benefit from homeopathic treatment, while women with menstrual or menopausal problems can also experience positive benefit.'

Beth MacEoin

The patient's view

'I first went to Beth MacEoin because I'd been feeling really unwell for some time. I'd been to my doctor, who said I was suffering from depression. My husband was working abroad at the time and only came home once a year, and I had two young children to bring up on my own. I felt really, really bad. I cried and shouted a lot, and felt as if I was in a black hole.

'I went to Beth as a last resort, and remember my first visit very well. I thought "What am I doing here?" I was incoherent and rambling, and thought "Why does she want to know the answer to these strange questions?" You couldn't get more sceptical than me, but I eventually went away with the little white tablets, and decided to give it a try.

'So I was amazed when it actually worked! From the first time I took the remedy I really started to feel different. There were small changes right from the beginning, I stopped crying as much, and felt better in myself.

'The changes were ongoing. I had suffered from urinary and chest infections whilst I was so down, but as I went on with homeopathy the antibiotics were left in the cupboard.

'Then I thought if it could do this for me, what could it do for my son

Christopher? He had been diagnosed with asthma at 3 years of age, and eczema since birth, which was always worse in hot weather. His quality of life was deeply affected.

'I decided to take him to Beth. Again homeopathy worked very well, and very quickly. He didn't need his inhaler though Beth advised me he should keep it with him. Now at 8 years of age, although he is affected if it is a particularly hot day for instance, he doesn't scratch and doesn't need his inhaler. Again I was amazed homeopathy worked so noticeably and steadily.

'Then my daughter Gillian burned her foot with boiling water about a year ago. Beth gave her remedies to assist the healing process, as we felt the wounds were healing too slowly. Not only did this quicken the process, but Gillian doesn't even have a scar.

'Although I would always go to Beth first now, none of us have been to her for about a year, as we have all been so well. She is approachable; if I haven't got an appointment she is happy to talk to and advise me by telephone, and I can pick up the remedies when I am passing. My own doctor is very good, but I have always felt hurried during consultations.

'It has been of great benefit to my family to have found something and someone I can rely on to provide alternative and effective treatment. I can recommend it!'

Anne Miller

Hypnotherapy

Origins

It is thought the ancient Greeks used a rudimentary form of hypnosis, and it has been practised in various ways throughout history, especially in religious and superstitious contexts. Modern hypnosis, however, was established by the Viennese physician, Franz Mesmer, in the late eighteenth century following his successful treatment of patients through the use of deep trance-like states. Mesmer's problem was that he never had the backing of his orthodox medical colleagues, and it took the more rational approach of a French country doctor by the name of Ambroise Liebeault to endow hypnotherapy with any kind of clinical credibility. He never claimed to possess any supernatural powers, and his explanation of what hypnotherapy could achieve was very much in keeping with our current understanding.

James Braid brought the practice to Britain in the late nineteenth century, and he used hypnotherapy in conjunction with his surgical practice. It was Braid who popularized the term 'hypnotism', derived from the Greek *hypnos*, meaning sleep. Unfortunately, stage hypnosis, which often held victims up to ridicule for the entertainment of others, earned medical hypnosis itself a bad name, and, was never truly accepted by the orthodox medical fraternity until 1955, when the British Medical Association finally acknowledged that it had a genuine place in the treatment of a number of clinical conditions.

Today, hypnotherapy is conducted within the NHS by doctors and psychologists, and it is sometimes used by non-medically qualified personnel, like the well-known Paul McKenna for example, who are able to help people in all sorts of ways. Hypnosis can help people overcome addictions to cigarettes, alcohol and other drugs and it can ease stress-related conditions which can seriously affect patients' general quality of life. Despite continued suspicion amongst some members of the medical profession, hypnosis has now become one of the most scientifically accepted of all the complementary therapies.

What is hypnosis?

Contrary to popular belief, hypnosis is not a state of deep sleep. It does involve the induction of a trance-like condition, but when in it, the patient is actually in an enhanced state of awareness, concentrating entirely on the hypnotist's voice. In this state, the conscious mind is suppressed and the subconscious mind is revealed. The therapist is able to suggest ideas, concepts and lifestyle adaptations to the patient, the seeds of which become firmly planted.

The practice of promoting healing or positive development in any way is known as hypnotherapy. As such, hypnotherapy is a kind of psychotherapy. The difference between hypnotherapy and normal psychotherapy, however, is that under hypnosis patients are generally much more suggestible and likely to accept guidance than they would ordinarily be. Hypnotherapy aims to reprogramme patterns of behaviour within the mind, enabling irrational fears, phobias, negative thoughts and suppressed emotions to be overcome. As the body is released from conscious control during the relaxed trance-like state of hypnosis, breathing becomes slower and deeper, the pulse rate drops and the metabolic rate falls. Similar changes along nervous pathways and hormonal channels enable the sensation of pain to become less acute, and the awareness of unpleasant symptoms, such as nausea or indigestion, to be alleviated.

How does it work?

Hypnosis is thought to work by altering our state of consciousness in such a way that the analytical left-hand side of the brain is turned off, whilst the non-analytical right-hand side is made more alert. The conscious control of the mind is inhibited, and the subconscious mind awoken. Since the subconscious mind is a deeper-seated, more instinctive force than the conscious mind, this is the part which has to change for the patient's behaviour and physical state to alter. For example, a patient who consciously wants to overcome their fear of spiders may try everything they consciously can to do it, but will still fail as long as their subconscious mind retains this terror and prevents the patient from succeeding. Progress can only be made by reprogramming the subconscious so that deep-seated instincts and beliefs are abolished or altered.

Is hypnotherapy effective?

If hypnosis were not effective, dentists would give up using the technique to reduce their patients' pain during procedures, and oncologists (cancer specialists) would no longer ask hypnotherapists to help their terminally ill patients to overcome discomfort and apprehension, and the nausea and sickness engendered by radiotherapy or chemotherapy. Many patients with irritable bowel syndrome have reported improvements after hypnosis, and Dr Peter Whorwell, a gastroenterologist and Director of Medicine at Manchester's Withington Hospital, reports a very high success rate amongst this patients treated with the technique. Not only did his patients' symptoms improve, but some even became symptom free and stayed that way for several months after therapy was discontinued. Other studies have shown hypnotherapy to be useful during childbirth, reducing the need for painkillers and actually making delivery itself quicker. Other studies, published in the *American Journal of Clinical Hypnosis*, have suggested that the duration of warts on the skin and the pain from burns can be reduced. Still more work has confirmed the benefits of the technique in helping some patients to give up smoking, and others to learn to live with tinnitus (a perpetual ringing, buzzing or hissing noise in the ear). A few people can be hypnotized into a very deep trance and have even undergone surgical operations using nothing other than this technique. This, however, has usually only been carried out in experimental settings, and it has no real practical use as a routine form of anaesthesia.

What form might the treatment take?

Firstly, any misconceptions a potential patient may have about hypnosis should be dispelled. The technique does not involve the patient being put into a deep sleep, and the patient cannot be made to do anything they would not ordinarily do. They remain fully aware of their surroundings and situation, and are not vulnerable to every given command of the therapist. The important thing is that the patient wants to change some behavioural habit or addiction and is highly motivated to do so. They have to want the treatment to work and must establish a good clinical rapport with the therapist in order for it to do so.

The first consultation may last for up to an hour or an hour and half during which the patient is asked what it is that has brought them to the clinic, what they wish to achieve, and what their understanding is of the technique. Any misconceptions or queries are addressed at this stage. The patient is then encouraged to relax in a comfortable environment where distractions are unlikely, preferably in a chair or on a couch. The therapist does *not* then dangle a watch on a chain in front of the patient's eyes, but will use a simple device in order to focus the patient's eyes on a fixed point. He or she may, for example, ask the patient to look at a spot on the ceiling. The patient is then encouraged to breathe slowly and deeply and to close their eyes and is then taken through a short routine which suggests that the eyelids are becoming heavier and heavier or that the arms are becoming so heavy that they cannot be lifted. A deep sigh often signals the onset of the hypnotic induction, following which suggestion therapy can take place.

While the patient is under hypnosis, the therapist offers guidance on how to overcome emotional difficulties, stresses or anxieties, and suggests ways of overcoming addictions or other bad or antisocial habits. The therapist can, for example, plant the idea in the subconscious mind that the sight of another cigarette will make the patient physically nauseated so they will never want to light up another. By encouraging the patient with a phobia to envisage in their mind a calm and relaxing scene whenever they encounter the object of their phobia, they can, through repeated therapy, marry the phobia with the calming scenario so that the two cancel each other out. Similarly, the athlete who always comes third in a race because they do not truly believe they can win can have positive images implanted in their subconscious mind which enable them initially to visualize breaking the winning tape first, and eventually to overcome their defeatist attitude and surpass their limiting expectations.

'Hypnohealing', a modern variant of hypnosis, is not practised by all hypnotherapists and is a technique designed to overcome physical ailments. Linked to the relatively new science of psycho-neuro-immunology, hypnohealers encourage patients to visualise the immune cells in their bodies rallying against and defeating diseased, inflammatory or malignant cells, in an attempt to overcome pathological processes. Whether it really works or not remains to be seen, but it is encouraged in many of Britain's

NHS hospitals and at the very least it changes a patient's attitudes from one of complete passivity to active resistance against illness.

The readiness and ability of patients to be hypnotized varies considerably and hypnotherapy generally requires several sessions in order to achieve meaningful results. However, the patient can learn the technique of self-hypnosis, which can be practised at home, to reinforce the usefulness of formal sessions with the therapist. This can help counter distress and anxiety-related conditions.

At the very end of a session, the therapist gently brings the patient back to full consciousness, using a recognized verbal device. This will be something along the lines of 'When I count backwards from 3 to 2 to 1 to 0 you will wake, relaxed, refreshed and alert.' Fears that patients sometimes have that they will not be properly brought out of hypnosis are unfounded

What problems are helped by hypnotherapy?

Hypnotherapy can be applied to many psychological, emotional and physical disorders. It is used to relieve pain in surgery and dentistry and has proved to be of benefit in obstetrics. It can shorten the delivery stage of labour and reduce the need for painkillers. It can ease the suffering of the disabled and those facing terminal illness, and it has been shown to help people to overcome addictions such as smoking and alcoholism, and to cope with bulimia. Children are generally easy to hypnotize and can be helped with nocturnal enuresis (bedwetting) and chronic asthma, whilst teenagers can conquer stammering or blushing problems which can otherwise make their lives miserable. Phobias of all kinds lend themselves well to hypnotherapy, and anyone suffering from panic attacks or obsessional compulsive behaviour, and stress-related problems like insomnia, may benefit. Conditions exacerbated by tension, such as irritable bowel syndrome, psoriasis and eczema, and excessive sweating, respond well, and even tinnitus and clicky jaws (tempero-mandibular joint dysfunction) can be treated by these techniques.

Is it safe?

Salacious newspaper headlines claiming that patients have not been properly brought out of a hypnotic trance and have gone on to commit antisocial acts quite out of character have not been substantiated. Also, those very rare cases where disreputable or unqualified 'therapists' have sexually abused women under hypnosis have been unfairly blown up out of all proportion. Stage hypnosis has alarmed many because it holds people up to ridicule, but this is not what hypnotherapy itself is about. In the hands of registered, properly qualified therapists who are members of established organizations, hypnosis is very safe and can be practised on everyone, including children as young as four.

How can I find a hypnotherapist?

Although anybody can freely advertise themselves as hypnotherapists, the best way to find a good one is to contact either the British Society of Medical and Dental Hypnosis or the British Society of Experimental and Clinical Hypnosis. Their members are all doctors, psychologists or dentists who have had subsidiary training in hypnosis. There are many thousands of hypnotherapists who are not registered with either of these organizations, and many have put unrecognized initials after their name. A few have only picked up the basic technique of hypnosis over a weekend or two. Lay hypnotists can be very effective, however, and those with the letters REG.HYP (Registered Hypnotherapist) or AC.HYP (Accredited Hypnotherapist) or N-SHAP (Graduate of the National School of Hypnotherapy and Psychotherapy) are amongst them. The real skill of a good therapist is knowing how to suggest the correct guidance to patients once they have been hypnotized in order to bring about clinical improvement. When looking for a therapist, ask your family doctor first if he or she can recommend someone locally; if not, contact one of the main organizations.

How much will it cost?

You should be able to find treatment costing no more than £50–60 per hour. Overcoming mild addictions should be achievable within a few weeks, but chronic deep-seated phobias or panic attacks will obviously require more frequent treatment.

The sceptic's view

The cynic can point to hundreds of thousands of patients who have spent a lot of money being hypnotized in order to quit smoking, only to return to the habit in a bigger way when the money has been spent. The benefit may last for a few weeks (as treatment often does when you have forked out hard cash for it), but the effects are short-lived. Hypnotists themselves say that patients cannot be made to do things they would not ordinarily do, so why should it help them to overcome habits when ordinarily they cannot do this *without* hypnosis? It is an interesting phenomenon, and an amusing turn when carried out in a West End theatre, but as a serious adjunct to conventional therapy it is really rather wacky. It may well be able to reduce the need for painkillers by relaxing people and allaying their fears, but you cannot perform major operations with it, and it often leaves patients deeply suspicious of what has happened to them in one of these trances. Perhaps the technique is best left to psychiatrists.

The therapist's view

'Although many cases of irritable bowel syndrome (IBS) respond to a combination of dietary changes and medication, a substantial proportion of patients continue to suffer considerably despite all the efforts of the doctor. In 1982, we decided to see if hypnotherapy could help a group of people and proved in a 'clinic trial' that it is highly effective. Since that time, we have treated hundreds of patients with an overall success rate of approximately 70 per cent. Patients with severe IBS have a terrible quality of life, and many are permanently off work because of their problem. In more recent studies we have shown that both these aspects of the problem are also helped by hypotherapy, with many people being able to resume employment.

'One of the most interesting aspects of our research in this area is that we have shown that the abnormalities that are present in the bowel of patients with IBS are put right by this form of treatment, thus proving that hypnotherapy does not just help anxiety or give a patient a psychological boost. It seems that it can actually rectify bodily functions that have gone wrong.'

Dr Peter J. Whorwell
Consultant Physician and Senior Lecturer in Medicine, University of Manchester

The patient's view

'I suffered terribly for many years with agoraphobia and panic attacks. I used to get into such a state about having to go shopping that it made me physically sick with worry. It got to the point that I developed sweaty palms, a feeling of nausea and palpitations just having to go down the garden path to collect my letters from the mail box. My doctor told me it was so socially disabling that I required antidepressants and tranquillizers. But these only made me worse; they made me feel like a zombie and I had similar panic attacks at the mere thought of having to do anything when I hadn't got the tablets with me. Eventually I was referred for hypnotherapy which, within six weeks, gave me a new lease of life. I learned to self-hypnotize and could reduce any feelings of panic as soon as I felt them welling up inside me whenever I was in a crowded place away from home. A neighbour of mine also had hypnotherapy to help give up smoking and it worked for her as well. I would heartily recommend this form of alternative therapy to anyone with problems like ours.'

Andrea Richards

Iridology

Origins

Examination of the eye as a method of general diagnosis goes back thousands of years and is an essential part of the full clinical examination carried out by orthodox doctors today. However, iridology itself was born in the nineteenth century by Ignatz Von Peczely (1826–1911), who came to believe that detailed examination of the iris alone, as opposed to the whole of the eye, could detect individual vulnerability to ill-health and any tendency or susceptibility to disease. The story goes that whilst playing with an owl, Von Peczely accidentally broke the bird's leg as he tried to withdraw his arm from it's sharp claws. At the very moment the owl's leg was fractured, Von Peczely apparently noticed a black streak appear in one of the owl's eyes. Many years later, when he was working as a homeopath, he was struck by a similar marking in the eye of a patient with a broken leg. He examined the eyes of several of his patients and came to the conclusion that his patients' diseases and the markings in their eyes were closely correlated. Eventually he drew up complete maps of the eye, identifying which regions of the iris were associated with particular organs elsewhere in the body, and he published his findings in 1880. Over the years, these iridology maps have been further progressed and refined, and are sometimes used by contemporary practitioners of iridology to help in the diagnosis of both psychological and physical disorders in patients.

What is iridology ?

Iridology simply refers to the examination of the iris of the eye to assess a patient's health and their susceptibility to any emotional or physical ailments. It uses iris charts which have been developed over the years from their early origins in the nineteenth century, but it in no way parallels the established and respected science of ophthalmology, which examines every aspect of the eye as well as the iris, and has no anatomical or physiological basis in common with ophthalmology. Reputable iridologists will always advise patients in whom they discover a weakness or developing susceptibility to disease to consult their GP as they do not regard iridology as a substitute for conventional diagnosis, merely as a complementary and additional technique.

How does it work?

By examining the iris of each eye in detail for markings, shadows, spots and colours, the iridologist attempts to assess the condition of a patient's health, both generally and specifically in each major organ of the body. Each iris is divided radially into 12 different sections, with each section representing part of the body, such as the large intestine, the thyroid gland, the liver or skin. There are also circular zones, representing certain systems in the body, such as the circulation and lymphatic channels, and by and large, the structures on the right-hand side of the body are featured in the right iris, and those on the left-hand side of the body, in the left iris.

Is iridology effective?

Ophthalmologists routinely examine their patients' irises as part of their screening examination of the eyes, because the irises can reveal disorders such as glaucoma and nervous system abnormalities. However, ophthalmologists do not subscribe to the claims of iridologists and do not accept that iridology has any place in modern medicine. They do not examine the texture and colour of the iris, and do not believe that its features can change or that its permanent and unalterable markings have anything to do whatsoever with the condition of the body's internal organs. The iris is of most interest to the ophthalmologist in showing signs of cholesterol deposits which may be laid down in a concentric ring around the margin of the iris, and in the ability of the iris to contract and expand in reaction to light shining through the pupil. Consultant ophthalmologists and opticians have seen numerous patients who have been incorrectly diagnosed by iridologists, and the clinical studies used by iridologists to support their work are usually based on the well-known finding of cholesterol deposits at the margins of the irises in patients with known high blood cholesterol levels. One famous study carried out in Maastricht by the Professor of Epidemiology at the University of Limberg showed very clearly that iridologists were no better at diagnosing gall bladder disease than anybody doing it by pure guess-work. Not only were their diagnoses no more correct than one could expect by chance, but the iridologists were also unable to tell just by looking at their patients' eyes, which patients had known and documented disease and which were absolutely healthy.

What form might the treatment take?

The average length of a first consultation with an iridologist is one hour. The patients' eyes will be examined with a small torch and a magnifying glass, and some practitioners will use a special camera with a macro-lens to make a photographic slide of the irises so they can be shown on a video screen in magnified form. The practitioner may well make notes as he studies the colour and clarity of the patient's irises and it is possible that he or she will recommend changes they think should be made to the patient's lifestyle or diet. Some iridologists also practise other forms of complementary therapy, such as naturopathy or homeopathy, and they may suggest treatment accordingly.

What problems are helped by iridology?

Iridologists claim that they can detect any innate susceptibility to important diseases such as arthritis or heart disease, and that they can detect poor kidney function or sluggish digestion.

Is it safe?

Iridology should be entirely safe for anybody in whatever state of health and at any age. Certainly, having a photograph taken of your eyes and having the irises looked at by an iridologist using a small torch can do no lasting physical damage. The danger of iridology, however, arises when it is used as an alternative to conventional diagnosis, leading to a real disorder being missed and neglected. Many people have taken up iridology with no qualifications whatsoever, and their advice is of no more use than that of an astrologer. For those people who are intrigued and charmed by having their irises read, the real danger exists that they will set too much store by an iridologist's conclusions, which have no foundation in scientific fact.

How can I find an iridologist?

Iridology is completely unregulated in the UK, but there are two organizations which have drawn up a code of conduct and ethics and can provide names and addresses of registered practitioners. The first is the Guild of Naturopathic Iridologists who have about 70 practitioners on their books, all of whom have permission to attach the letters RIr after their names. The second organization is the International Association of Clinical Iridologists, whose graduates have studied at their own college of iris analysis, and are then eligible for the title of MCIrA.

How much will it cost?

Patients can expect to pay about £40 for the first appointment, which for most people will be a one-off diagnostic session.

The sceptic's view

When confronted with the origins of iridology the sceptic might reasonably say that anyone clumsy enough to break a wild bird's leg whilst playing with it is not cut out to become a member of the caring professions in the first place! He might also point out how convenient it is that the right-hand side of the body is represented in the right eye and vice versa. If only all anatomical observation were that easy. The truth is that the characteristics of the iris do not change in response to internal disease; ironically it is about the only part of the eye that does not. The retina at the back of the eye changes in cases of high blood pressure or in diabetes and even in the presence of a brain tumour, and the white of the eye, the sclera at the front, will turn yellow in the presence of jaundice, but the iris, alas, is the least useful bit of the eye to observe for diagnostic purposes. Iridologists have simply chosen it since the irises are at the centre of facial expression and sexual attraction, and people have long been fascinated by the eyes being the 'windows of the soul'. Convenient, too, the sceptic might think, that the circular irises resemble clock faces, as they are divided into 12 sections by the iridologist. Scientific studies have shown iridology to be of no more benefit than guess-work, so the disbeliever would need a great deal of persuasion ever to accept iridology as being of any use whatsoever to even the most gullible patient.

The therapist's view

'Iridology offers a quick, non-invasive and painless system of health analysis through the iris of the eye. The irises reveal hereditary tendencies, and genetic strengths and weaknesses, as well as the strength of individual organs. For instance, hyperacidity in the stomach, spastic colon, congestion in the lungs, hardening of the arteries, underfunctioning kidneys, poor circulation and an overactive thyroid gland are just a few of literally hundreds of conditions identified through an examination of the irises.

'Changes in the appearance of the iris – the lines, flecks and pigments – all reflect how the various tissues in the body are functioning. The iris is concerned only with the state of the tissue (e.g. acidity, toxicity, lymphatic congestion, hardened arteries, weak lung tissue, accumulated tension, degenerated tissues, etc.). However, it is important to note that the iris does not reveal specific pathology because many diseases cause similar changes in body tissue. It is, therefore, not a substitute for conventional forms of diagnosis, but rather a very valuable complementary tool.

'Iridology is therefore both positive and preventative – a thorough form of holistic health analysis helping to identify and treat the underlying cause(s) of any health problems rather than focusing on the symptoms alone. It is a unique complementary diagnostic tool and is therefore appropriate whenever the underlying root cause of a health problem needs to be identified. However, one of the best features and main advantages of Iridology over other forms of health analysis is that changes are said to appear in the iris before the physical symptom develops. This enables preventative action to be taken to improve health and avoid those diseases which might otherwise follow. For example, one marking – a white-yellow arc around the periphery of the iris, commonly known as an "arcus senilis" – has been said by iridologists, for centuries, to be indicative, of hardening of the arteries. Recent research in the US has shown that nine out of ten people who have this marking have high serum cholesterol levels and are more than twice as likely to suffer with heart disease than people who do not have this marking.

'Although not yet fully accepted by conventional medicine, iridology is commonly used by doctors in Europe, Australasia and North America, and it is rapidly becoming one of the most popular forms of complementary medicine.'

Adam J. Jackson

The patient's view

'I've always been a bit cynical about doctors in hospitals and I've experimented with lots of complementary therapies over the years. When I saw an iridologist out of interest he spent over an hour carefully examining my eyes and told me he believed I had a weakness in one of my kidneys. This was news to me so I had it checked out. It turned out that I had a mild infection in my bladder which I was not aware of; and had this been neglected it might well have spread upwards to my kidneys and caused a very serious infection called pyelonephritis. I had a course of antibiotics, religiously drank several litres of water every day to flush the system through, and (touch wood) have never had any lasting trouble. I certainly believe there is something in iridology, and that more people ought to consider trying it.'

Lesley Goodman

Macrobiotics

Origins

The word 'macrobiotics' is derived from two Greek words, *makros*, meaning large, and *bios*, meaning life. According to the basic macrobiotic philosophy, we can only remain healthy by striking a balance with the environment that surrounds us, and of which we are an integral part. Macrobiotics originated in early Tibet and China, and was first documented in three well-known books, namely *The Nei Ching*, *The I Ching* and *The Tao Te Ching*.

The fundamental concept of Yin and Yang ran throughout the three books, the tenet being that there are two equal and opposite forces in nature which interact with one another, and between which there must always be balance and equilibrium. Yin represents that which is fluid, cool and flexible, whereas Yang represents that which is hot, dynamic and potent. Yin and Yang can be found in everything, every object and every biological cycle, and human beings themselves are made up of elements of Yin and Yang. Yin characteristics are those represented by a relaxed and laid-back attitude, a calm demeanour, and a penchant for creativity and sociability. Yang characteristics, on the other hand, include vigour, an alert and focused mind, attention to detail and busy activity. The macrobiotic therapist believes that illness and poor health result from either Yin or Yang being dominant over the other. Excess Yang can lead to stress, irritability, tension, insomnia, palpitations, weight loss and hyperactivity. Excess Yin can lead to feeling tired all the time, lassitude and even depression and weight gain.

The macrobiotic philosophy holds that Yin and Yang can be influenced by many factors in our lives, including the way we operate within our environment, exercise and diet. Macrobiotic therapists these days tend to concentrate on the work of George Ohsawa, who condensed thousands of years of ancient macrobiotic philosophy into a more comprehensive form of nutritional therapy, and who claimed that by altering the balance of foods within a person's diet it was possible to counter illness and prevent disease. On this basis, somebody increasing their dietary intake of Yin foods could feel better if they were suffering from too much Yang. Conversely, somebody feeling the effect of too much Yin, could increase their intake of Yang foods and experience the benefits. Ohsawa was influenced by the work of a Japanese doctor called Sagen Ishizuka who, in the 1880s came to the conclusion that a diet consisting largely of whole grains and vegetables and devoid of refined carbohydrates and white rice could prevent disease. Ohsawa condensed his own beliefs with those of the more ancient macrobiotic philosophy, and in 1945 coined the modern term 'macrobiotics'.

A student of Ohsawa's, Michio Kushi, began teaching the macrobiotic philosophy in Europe and the USA in the 1960s. He broadened Ohsawa's original ideas even further and his teachings became of great interest to many. The concept that anyone can derive the best out of life by using dietary means to promote physical, psychological and emotional health is obviously appealing.

What is macrobiotics?

Macrobiotic therapy is a combination of philosophy, lifestyle and diet. The philosophy tells us that macrobiotics works by preventing disease rather than correcting problems that have already arisen. The recommended lifestyle attempts to ensure that everyone lives each day to the full in perfect harmony and happiness, avoiding negative thoughts, emotions and concepts as much as possible. A healthy lifestyle should be based on happy family dynamics, a sociable approach to other people and the generation of a wide circle of friends among whom no prejudice exists and the ability to share and to show kindness, compassion and support to others is encouraged. The diet itself has been likened to that of a Japanese peasant and breaks down in the following way:

- 50 per cent cooked whole grain pasta, bread, rice or noodles;
- 25 per cent vegetables prepared in a variety of ways;
- 10 per cent protein derived from fish, pulses or soya bean products such as cheese (tofu) or tempeh;
- 5 per cent sea vegetables prepared in soups or stews;
- 5 per cent soups of fish, beans or other vegetables;
- 5 per cent teas and desserts which can consist of seeds or nuts, fermented rice or fruit.

Some macrobiotic regimes are stricter than others but, generally, sugar, spices and alcohol, which are thought to be influenced by Yin factors are discouraged, and eggs, cheese and meat, thought to be dominated by excess Yang are also discouraged. Therapists believe these foodstuffs have a potent effect on the human organism and can imbalance its system, leading to illness.

How does it work?

A macrobiotic practitioner will attempt to balance energy flow within the body by adjusting diet accordingly. Foods that might be used effectively to increase Yin include: green leafy vegetables; seeds and nuts; tofu and tempeh; whole fruit; fruit and vegetable juices; jams (organically made); barley malt. Yang foods include: whole grain cereals such as brown rice, wholemeal bread, wholemeal flour and oats; root vegetables such as turnips, parsnips and potatoes; fish and shellfish; protein-containing beans, peas and lentils; salt; soya bean products.

Macrobiotic practitioners often tell their patients that when they change to a macrobiotic diet they will notice improvements in their health within 10 days. This is based on the belief that the fluid in the blood (plasma) in which the red and white cells are suspended, and which forms about half of the blood volume, is renewed every 10 days. Since they believe the plasma is directly influenced by macrobiotic nutrition, patients are told they will notice physical changes in themselves after that time. These changes may include unpleasant symptoms such as insomnia, tension, irritability and fatigue as well as cravings for strong flavoured foods which people have become accustomed to over the years. Gradually, however, many patients start to feel better in themselves with sharper and more focused concentration, a spring in their step and a calmer and more balanced outlook on life.

Therapists will claim that even people with chronic disorders can experience obvious improvement within a few weeks. No therapist pretends that it is easy to change to a macrobiotic diet, but reliance on it can be learned and established within as little as three weeks. It has been shown that devotees of macrobiotics are able to stick to their unique diet quite effortlessly once they have mastered the principles.

Is macrobiotics effective?

It is difficult to prove scientifically that a nutritional therapy which incorporates lifestyle changes and the adoption of a new philosophy can genuinely improve a person's health. It has not been the subject of clinical research, partly because it is difficult to separate the possible beneficial consequences of reducing a patient's stress levels and altering their sedentary lifestyle whilst at the same time altering their diet. But macrobiotic practitioners, however, have converted hundreds of people to their way of life, and these disciples adhere rigidly to their new *modus vivendi*. Certainly, with all the medical problems associated with our frenetic and rather antisocial world with its over reliance on highly processed refined foods, there is a lot to recommend it. Also, given the enormous difficulties that a huge proportion of our population have in losing weight, exercising and making their way socially in the world, perhaps many could benefit from the fairly disciplined approach of modern macrobiotics.

What form might the treatment take?

Macrobiotic practitioners diagnose in much the same way as acupuncturists or practitioners of Chinese herbal medicine. During a consultation, the patient would have their eyes, face, tongue and hands examined, and all the time the therapist would be listening to the sound of the patient's voice and assessing the content of what they were saying in order to ascertain their nature and personality as well as the balance of Yin and Yang within them. The pulses on the inside of both wrists would be palpated, and of course a full medical history would be taken, including details of the patient's exercise habits, lifestyle, diet and current symptoms. Dietary recommendations would then be given, suggesting which foods should be avoided for up to 30 days, and which foodstuffs should be taken in preference. Sometimes herbal decoctions or teas are prescribed to supplement the new diet. The recommendations are usually founded on Michio Kushi's standard macrobiotic diet, although adjustments and refinements are made according to the individual's needs. Consultations usually last about an hour, and at least two sessions are needed to pinpoint the diet correct for the individual.

What problems are helped by macrobiotics?

The most enthusiastic followers of macrobiotics claim that it is capable of preventing disease from occurring in the first place. This is, of course, difficult to prove, as is the tenet that macrobiotics can boost the immune system. Broadly speaking, however, the three-pronged approach of macrobiotics is theoretically capable of helping people overcome difficulties in their social, emotional, spiritual and physical lives, whilst being able to reduce symptoms within the digestive, nervous and hormonal systems. It helps people to lose weight where necessary, to increase their energy levels, to enhance their concentration, and also to build up muscular strength and stamina. Many people with chronic illness, such as rheumatism, eczema and even some types of cancer, have experienced improvement in their symptoms as a result of adopting this therapy.

Is it safe?

These days, macrobiotic diets broadly encompass contemporary scientific thinking about what constitutes sensible, balanced nutrition. Consequently macrobiotics, as practised by registered practitioners, is generally safe for most sections of society. Formerly, as recently as the 1970s and 1980s, potentially hazardous types of macrobiotic diet were being recommended, which involved the consumption of brown rice and precious little else. As a result, severe malnutrition was reported in both adults and children, which, at the time, brought the philosophy of macrobiotics a bad name. More recently, however, microbiotics has enjoyed another surge in popularity and is generally considered safe, although it is always advisable that the patient's orthodox doctor is consulted before this therapy is begun. Once this is done, even pregnant and breast feeding women, and children can adopt a macrobiotic diet, providing it is not too strict and restrictive. The diet, of course, should always be tailored to the patient's individual requirements.

How can I find a practitioner?

Qualified registered practitioners of macrobiotics will come under the auspices of the Kushi Institute, based in the USA, and will have studied there for at least two years. There is always the risk that a patient seeing anyone else who claims to be a practitioner but who is not registered with the Institute may end up being given an unbalanced and nutritionally incorrect diet which could do them much more harm than good. Always check with your own GP about any change to your ordinary diet.

How much will it cost?

An hour's consultation will cost somewhere in the region of £40.

The sceptic's view

The cynic would hold macrobiotics up as another example of a trendy therapy that offers nothing new whilst being potentially capable of causing harm. In fact, a decade or two ago, macrobiotics was creating a great deal of harm by producing severe malnutrition in many groups in society who were too stupid or gullible to know any better. It is surely obvious that if people adjusted their lifestyle to take more exercise and eat less fat, then we would not have a problem with obesity in society, heart disease rates would fall, and people would feel generally better. We do not need a macrobiotic therapist, trained in some fancy American institute, to tell us that we should stop smoking and eat a healthier and more natural diet. As for the Yin and Yang concept, it is all very imaginative but we already have a much better way of discovering which foods contain most energy since nutritional values are now clearly printed on the sides of most food packets, and they tell us in precise numerical terms what we need to know. Since the human alimentary canal can only recognize the basic components of food in terms of their calorific value, the sceptic has little time for Yin and Yang. The sceptic feels able to determine with confidence exactly how to live his or her own life, and which foods should and should not be eaten, without having to pay £40 for the privilege.

The therapist's view

We are what we eat, and even the most erudite and academic of scientists these days will agree that many forms of illness and disease, including cancer are directly related to diet. Unfortunately, this does not stop people dying from and suffering from these diseases, and therefore millions of people could benefit from dietary adjustment and lifestyle changes as recommended by someone qualified to propose them.

Macrobiotic therapy is satisfying in that all aspects of a person's life are taken into account, and the approach is entirely holistic. Coupled with the fact that thousands of people with acute and chronic illnesses have derived benefit as well as the countless thousands who have been prevented from falling ill in the first place, the rewards for both patient and therapist are immeasurable. Rather than being a therapy which is likely to be phased out as a result of further advances in modern medicine, macrobiotics is probably destined to become increasingly popular.

The patient's view

'When I was first introduced to a macrobiotics therapist I had just ended a tempestuous relationship. I felt absolutely exhausted, my concentration was lousy, I had no energy or stamina and no desire to do very much about it. I think my best friend felt sorry for me, and because she had enormous faith in her therapist, she dragged me along to share the experience. Two years down the line and I have to say this has turned my life around. Every day of my life is different now in that I exercise, I eat carefully, I have more restful sleep and even my interests and my outlook on the environment have changed. I feel more in control, I feel vital and energized and whenever anyone ribs me about being somewhat obsessive about my new regime, I just say I don't care, because it works for me.'

Bonnie Blowers

Massage Therapy

Origins

Massage therapy may well be the oldest treatment known to humankind but it is likely that the instinctive cradling, touching, and stroking which we all employ in loving relationships were also employed by Neanderthal man. Massage was certainly used thousands of years ago by the Chinese, and references to massaging the skin with oil can be found in both the Bible and the Koran. The ancient Greeks and Romans used it to prepare their soldiers and gladiators for combat, and Hippocrates referred to it and prescribed it for his patients around 400 BC. He wrote 'The physician must be qualified in many things, but most assuredly in rubbing.'

Massage therapy was adopted in many cultures throughout the world as the human population evolved, but then in Europe, during the Middle Ages, it gradually came to be regarded as sinful. God-fearing churches felt it engendered physical and spiritual pleasure, and consequently it was roundly condemned. Thankfully, in the early nineteenth century, Per Henrik Ling, a Swedish gymnast, developed many therapeutic massages which collectively came to be known as Swedish massage, and went on to become the foundation of massage therapy today.

During the twentieth century, massage in all its various guises has come in and out of fashion. During the First World War it was used extensively in the physical and emotional rehabilitation of battle-wounded soldiers. By the Second World War, however, it was almost completely overshadowed by the staggering and rapid advances in medical technology and powerful pharmaceutical medications like penicillin and sulphonamide drugs. In the last 30 years, massage therapy has again found favour amongst members of the caring professions who are able to recognize its considerable benefits, and it is widely adopted today in NHS pain clinics, in residential accommodation for the elderly, in hospices, in cancer wards and in physiotherapy departments. Unfortunately, its reputation has been tarnished thanks to the tacky misuse of the word 'massage' by the sex industry and the escort agencies which abound throughout the world. 'Massage' is therefore understood by some to be a synonym for those services offered by prostitutes, which is extremely unfortunate since bona fide massage therapy has an established and useful role in modern medical practice.

What is massage therapy?

Massage therapy involves the physical application of touch to the soft tissues of the body to promote well-being and health. It is safe, relaxing and gentle, and because it involves touch between the therapist and the patient it is able to bring them closer together with an emotional and physical bond that is impossible to equal in any distant or remote way. For the chronically sick or disabled, for those who are terminally ill and for those who are socially cut off from the rest of civilization the spiritual and psychological benefits are enormous.

Although derived from the Greek word *massein* which means, literally, to knead, it involves many other types of touch as well as kneading, such as stroking or 'effleurage', wringing or 'petrissage', pressure application, percussion and pounding. Pummelling or knuckling are also used in massage. Depending on the type of massage used, practitioners might use their hands, elbows or even their feet to apply the therapy. Some forms of treatment are very gentle and soothing, whereas others are powerful, forceful and at times somewhat uncomfortable. Some are applied to the body as a whole and others focus on particular areas such as the head and neck. Some are conducted on a special couch, some on a mat on the floor. Some types simply apply manipulation to the muscles, others are applied to specific points such as acupressure points or 'marma' points, the latter being a feature of ayurvedic-based Marma Indian massage.

The type of massage that European patients are probably most familiar with is Swedish massage – the type that is mainly practised within sports centres and health clubs. Any knots that are discovered in the musculo-skeletal system are eased out using fluent stroking movements using the flat of the hands or the thumbs. Oriental massage, on the other hand, tends to focus more on specific body points. These massages often employ oils or creams and, in keeping with the holistically orientated philosophies of oriental medicine, the purpose of the therapy is to restore equilibrium and harmony so that soma and psyche are at one.

The main types of oriental massage to be had in Britain are Thai massage, Reiki, Tuina and Marma. Reiki is really a form of healing involving a gentle touch, whereby the therapist attempts to discover areas of the patient's body which possess low levels of energy so that an input of energy can be directed through their own hands into the patient's body. Tuina is used as an adjunct to traditional Chinese medicine and involves the therapist palpating, twisting and pushing the soft tissues of the body with their fingers, hands and knuckles. Thai massage is normally delivered with the patient lying on the floor, and the therapist will often use not only the hands but the elbows, feet and knees as well. A Marma massage is used in conjunction with Indian ayurvedic medicine and is applied to any of the 107 specific marma points which are thought to influence all of the body's internal organs and their functions.

How does it work?

All types of massage are based on similar underlying principles. On one level they are relaxing, soothing and pleasurable; on another level they bring the therapist in closer contact with the patient and can contribute towards building a trusting therapeutic relationship. The treatment can then be brought to bear superficially on the patient to ease specific points of tension or irritation around the body, or, in a deeper sense, to restore function and equilibrium to all the distant organs of the body for the promotion of the spiritual, physical and emotional well-being of the whole.

The effect of massage therapy on the emotions was investigated by the Austrian psychoanalyst Wilhelm Reich during the early part of the twentieth century. He was impressed by the degree of muscle tension which could result from unresolved anger, frustration or grief. He came to believe that by dispelling this muscle tension pent-up emotions could be freed, thereby relaxing mental turmoil and allowing the patient to psychologically blossom. Physiologists have described how muscles might release endorphins, the body's natural opiates, and so ease pain and feelings of anxiety or depression.

Is massage therapy effective?

Precisely how effective massage therapy may be remains to be seen as relatively few well-devised scientific trials supplying meaningful evidence have been carried out. However, researchers at Harvard Medical School found that when massage was used in conjunction with pre-operative counselling and advice, patients required less pain relief post-operatively and were discharged from hospital several days earlier than patients who were given the same information without the massage. Whether this effect was merely obtained through the relief of anxiety is irrelevant; the results speak for themselves. In 1995, the Institute of Cancer Research also found that massage reduced anxiety, promoted relaxation and alleviated symptoms in patients with terminal illness. Moreover, it appears from clinical studies that depression could be lifted with the use of massage and that the early morning waking and insomnia associated with this condition could also be improved. Many NHS hospitals are happy to employ the services of massage therapists for all types of patients: for those in children's wards, intensive care, or isolation wards; for sufferers of AIDS and heart attack victims in coronary care units; for people undergoing rehabilitation for strokes; even for newborn babies in incubators in special care baby units. Massage certainly has an important role to play in the treatment of all these patients.

What form might the treatment take?

What happens during a consultation with a massage therapist will depend on the type of massage that he or she practises, and the patient's general state of health. Most therapists will want to know what symptoms the patient is currently suffering from, what their general state of health is like, whether there have been any serious problems in the past, and whether any orthodox treatment is currently being used. The therapist is also likely to ask about the patient's lifestyle, exercise and diet. Massage is often avoided in patients with any inflammatory skin conditions such as generalized eczema or psoriasis, and patients are advised not to have a big meal within an hour or two before or after the massage. The patient may or may not be asked to undress, and essential oils, creams or powders may or may not be used.

In Swedish massage, the therapist usually starts on the back, working down to the legs, then, when the patient turns over, the chest, abdomen, shoulders and face are treated. Different types of massage will obviously involve different approaches, different positions and different specific techniques, and, after an hour or so, any of them can make the patient feel quite different. Some people feel light-headed and detached; others may feel totally relaxed or invigorated or sometimes even slightly low in spirits.

It is, of course, quite possible for patients to teach themselves massage of a simple kind, and then practise on a partner or another member of the family. This is how to do it:

1 Use a warm, quiet, dark room where there are no distractions.
2 Remove any watches or jewellery which could scratch the skin.
3 Expose the area to be massaged.
4 Make sure the skin is clear of infection or inflammation and that whatever pain there is is not made worse or does not spread to other areas when pressure is applied.
5 The person being massaged should lie on a firm, padded surface.
6 Ideally, use an aromatherapy massage oil (see page 118) so your hands can glide smoothly over the skin. A light vegetable oil or talcum powder could be used instead.
7 Pour no more than one teaspoonful of massage oil into the palm of one hand, and warm the oil by rubbing your hands together.

8 Begin with circular movements, moulding your hands to the shape of the body and maintaining a constant rhythm.
9 Keep one hand in contact with the skin at all times. If more oil is needed, pour a little on to the back of the massaging hand and continue stroking as you use your other hand to transfer the oil on to the recipient's skin.
10 Keep conversation to a minimum during the massage.
11 On small areas, use only thumb and fingertips.
12 On large areas, use the whole hand and firmer pressure.
13 If massage causes tickling, either increase the pressure or go on to different parts.
14 If muscle tone is being treated, the thumb should exert deep pressure, moving in small circles.
15 To release tension in muscles around the shoulder or pelvic girdle and thighs, a kneading technique can be used which involves pummelling with the edge of the hand to create a chopping, bouncing effect on the muscles.

What problems are helped by massage therapy?

Massage is particularly good at relieving fibrositis, a sluggish lymphatic system and any uncomfortable disorder of the musculo-skeletal system. It is able to dissipate anxiety, to prevent insomnia, and to improve general well-being in everyone, including the chronically disabled, the socially isolated and the terminally ill. Massage can be used in patients of all ages, with or without symptoms, and, according to some of the massage techniques used in older medical philosophies, can restore full healthy function to all parts of the body, not only restoring physiological activity, but also preventing the development of future disease.

Is it safe?

Generally speaking, massage is safe, but to reduce any possible side effects, patients with certain conditions should not be treated. These include women in the first trimester of pregnancy, patients with moderate varicose veins, thrombophlebitis (inflamed veins), and anyone with symptoms of nerve entrapment, blood clot or a temperature.

How can I find a massage therapist?

The basic answer is almost anywhere, but how to obtain a therapeutically useful massage is a more difficult question to answer. Since therapy is entirely unregulated in Britain, patients generally subject themselves to massage very much at their own risk. There is a bewildering abundance of massage qualifications, some obtained in a couple of weekends, others representing 2 years' hard graft. Although large numbers of colleges and training schools have been set up, there still remain no established educational curriculum and no minimum requirements of competence. The British Massage Therapy Council is attempting to set up a recognized register of reputable therapists, and the Massage Therapy Institute of Great Britain lists several hundred therapists, whose names can be supplied to applicants. At least 500 independent colleges run courses for people hoping to obtain International Therapy Examination Council qualifications (ITEC). If what the patient is looking for is a relaxing massage at the end of a busy week, or if the massage is part of basic beauty therapy, then it probably doesn't matter that the therapist only has minimal part-time training, but more significant medical conditions should always be treated by a skilled and experienced exponent of the art of good massage therapy. It is certainly not recommended that anyone find a therapist through advertisements in local newsagents or phone directories, and dubious-sounding offers of massage or personal services have little to do with any medically therapeutic treatment.

How much will it cost?

Most sessions will last between 30 minutes and 90 minutes, and the cost will vary according to the type of technique used.

Expect to pay a minimum of £15 and a maximum of £60. The majority of people will pay £20–25 per treatment.

The sceptic's view

Most people like to be touched because it feels good. It's a basic natural instinct for a human being to want to touch and to be touched, and of course this has a soothing and calming effect. For the socially isolated, this is more than welcome and probably has a greater effect than any known drug. However, this has nothing to do with medical therapy and is nothing more than a formalized type of close physical contact with a stranger, made acceptable by the fact that everyone colludes in the process. By all means supply it to children, pregnant women and the elderly in hospitals, cancer wards, special care units and residential accommodation, but please let us not pretend it is therapy; it is simply organized visiting with the laying on of hands. That there is no best way to do it is borne out by the fact that different so-called therapists will deliver the treatment in a variety of ways – some softly, some firmly, some even painfully. Because it remains unregulated, because anybody can quickly obtain some kind of massage qualification, and because it is widely known as a synonym for prostitution, massage therapy can never establish itself as a mainstream medical practice.

The therapist's view

'The wonderful thing about massage is that it is a powerful natural therapy which can be carried out at any time in the simplest environment with only a pair of caring hands. The therapist can learn a huge amount about the general state of health of the client from tension in muscles, skin type, texture, tone, colour changes, firm tissues, toned tissues and flabby tissues, and therefore can tailor the different movements to suit the client. Some techniques are deliberately stimulating, but in general the overall aim is to promote relaxation.

'It always gives me immense pleasure to work on a tense muscle and feel it soften and release under my hands.'

Phillippa Stacy, IFR
Tutor and Therapist

The patient's view

'I was overweight and over-stressed at work, and I wasn't happy with the way my life was going. I took up regular training and squash at a local health club, and although the weight came off my body felt stiff and sore the day after any training session. Loads of other people at the club were having massage therapy to physically and mentally relax them, and even the squash first team were in the habit of having sessions before games whenever they played a home match. A little nervously at first, I booked myself in for a few sessions, and I could not believe how beneficial it was. I feel a million dollars after each session, and I now move freely and easily the following day after even the hardest work-out. I will continue to have regular sessions whether or not I am using the gym in the future.'

Mark White

Meditation

Origins

Meditation was practised in Buddhist Monasteries as well as non-religious environments in Asia over 2,000 years ago. Transcendental meditation was developed and made famous by the Maharishi Mahesh Yogi in the 1960s, and was one of the many types of meditation ecstatically received by the flower power worshippers and hippies of that era. The Friends of the Western Buddhist Order, the FWBO, was established in Britain in 1967 and teaches meditation of a slightly different kind. Mantra meditation, as espoused by the School of Meditation, began in 1961, and this has familiarized thousands of patients with the technique. Consequently, large numbers of British people practise meditation on a daily basis, which involves sitting quietly for about 20 minutes twice a day. Many orthodox doctors use it as part of their clinical repertoire and the British Association for the Medical Application of Transcendental Meditation now boasts a membership of some 700 GPs and hospital physicians. In some parts of the world, meditation is so highly thought of as a preventative therapy that insurance companies allow regular meditators a discount on their private health insurance premiums.

What is meditation?

Not only is meditation useful in achieving spiritual awareness and fulfilment, but can also alleviate inner turmoil and achieve a state of deep relaxation by sweeping all thoughts and worries from the mind. It involves sitting comfortably in a quiet environment and focusing the mind on a neutral thought or object so that it becomes free to relax and find peace, happiness and fulfilment. Meditation is designed to improve physical, psychological and spiritual well-being, and it can be categorized into a number of different types.

Transcendental meditation

This type of meditation is usually used to reduce stress levels, and is often recommended by orthodox doctors. It now boasts some 200,000 followers in Britain and hundreds more are learning about TM every week. When sitting quietly, a personally significant word or 'mantra' is repeated in your head.

Buddhist meditation

A mantra, is not used in Buddhist meditation but instead the mind is focused on breathing techniques and on the abolition of negative feelings and their replacement by more positive and constructive thoughts. This form of meditation maintains that altered attitudes are necessary to eradicate destructive thought processes and emotions, and are the best way to achieve a greater sense of self-worth and spiritual contentment.

Mantra meditation

In Mantra meditation, as taught by the School of Meditation in London, the technique is centred on a basic word or sound, and the mind is allowed to drift without direction. In this way it is similar to TM. The individual is given a focal device or mantra which the meditator says over and over again to him or herself. The mantra is a personal secret word or sound which should have no emotional meaning whatsoever. The word could be 'om' or 'rah'. Some people prefer to use a word with a peaceful connotation such as 'ocean' or 'void'. Having chosen the focal device, the following steps are usually followed:

1 Choose a quiet environment where you will not be disturbed.
2 Take off your shoes and loosen all tight clothing. Sit in a comfortable position with your back straight.
3 Consciously 'let go' and be aware of the silence around you and the gentle ebb and flow of your breathing.
4 Breathe in and out gently through your nose.
5 As you breathe out, say the word 'rah' silently to yourself.
6 Breathe in again, then repeat 'rah' as you exhale.
7 Carry on doing this, concentrating only on your breathing and the repetition of the word 'rah'.
8 Clear your mind totally of all distractions.
9 If you find your mind wanders or that distracting thoughts start to intrude on your concentration, take yourself back to your breathing and the word 'rah'.
10 Meditate for 5 minutes at a time until you find it easy to clear your mind of all distractions.

With sufficient practice, the patient will gradually be able to increase their meditation time to up to 20 minutes. If possible, set aside a specific time every day to go through this technique as it will more than repay itself in terms of potential benefit. Often, the best time to do it is first thing in the morning or last thing at night. As Gandhi said, 'Meditation is the key to the morning, and the latch to the evening.'

How does it work?

Basically, there are two sides to the brain and each has a different function. In simple terms, the left side of the brain governs logic, analysis and word ability, and the right side of the brain governs creativity, fantasy, lateral thought, picture images and imagination. Unless you are meditating, it is only possible to use one side of the brain at a time. The left side of the brain normally dominates our consciousness, and when we repeat the one-word mantra during meditation, we occupy the left side of the brain with the monotonous job of concentrating on this. When we constantly bring our attention back to the focal device in this way, and away from all other distractions, the right side of the brain can then take over, resulting in the reduction of the stress response and a new-found freedom to relax. We feel a sense of tranquillity and serenity. This is borne out by recordings of brain-wave activity during meditation which show characteristic alpha rhythms closely associated with rest. Just like progressive and deep muscular relaxation, meditation can be practised anywhere suitable. However, anybody suffering from epilepsy or organic psychiatric disorders such as schizophrenia should consult their doctor before attempting meditation.

Is meditation effective?

That some people are able to rest and relax after meditation is not in question. The use of electroencephalograms (EEGs) during sessions of transcendental meditation has shown that alpha brain-waves (closely associated with rest) increase, but alterations to the blood supply to the skin and muscle tone also occur. Devotees maintain that they sleep better and are less anxious when they meditate regularly, and that they are able to reduce their smoking and drinking habits as a result. They feel that the benefits are accumulative and that the more meditation is practised the greater they can appreciate the effect it has on them. Hundreds of randomized controlled medical studies have been conducted on TM, in many different countries of the world, and most suggest that patients with anxiety, depression, sleeplessness, migraine, tension headache, irritable bowel syndrome, stomach ulcers, asthma and high blood pressure may all benefit.

Buddhists, however, do not pander to the need to prove scientifically that their therapy is effective. The FWBO claim that there are thousands of satisfied customers, a fact which speaks for itself. Interesting work carried out at the University of Massachusetts Medical Centre showed that long-term patients who, despite years of conventional treatment, had shown little improvement in their symptoms experienced a significant subjective improvement as well as a real boost to their self-confidence and the discovery of an inner peace after a mere two months of Buddhist-orientated meditation.

What form might the treatment take?

Since meditation requires a learned discipline, it is best to be taught the technique by a proper trainer. It is not a bad idea, however, to go to an initial lecture, read a booklet or even try a little meditation alone at home before committing time and money on a course.

Either individually or in a group, a newcomer to meditation will be shown how to sit comfortably, not necessarily cross-legged, but in an upright chair or sitting on their haunches with their feet placed under their pelvis. The arms should rest on the thighs or the lap, so that the shoulders are relaxed. The teacher will instruct pupils to concentrate on their breathing, telling them when to hold their breath and when to release it. The teacher may also suggest a mantra, or special word, or ask pupils to choose one for themselves. It can have religious connotation or it can simply have neutral or personal meaning.

An initial course in meditation usually involves sessions on a daily basis for up to a week, followed by another concentrated refresher course a few weeks later. Each session generally lasts for 1–2 hours.

What problems are helped by meditation?

Meditation is certainly useful for people who suffer from anxiety and tension. Any stress-related conditions, including palpitations, migraine, headaches, indigestion, nausea, irritable bowel syndrome, tremor and insomnia, respond well, but so do behavioural symptoms such as over-eating, excessive use of cigarettes and alcohol, constant irritability, suppressed anger, paranoia and general fatigue. Even sexual disorders, such as infertility, menstrual irregularities, impotence and reduced libido, may respond. Over and above the specific conditions, meditation is often reported to bring about greater self-esteem and general self-confidence.

Is it safe?

Meditation works in such a way that experimentation without the aid of a teacher can sometimes allow troublesome anxieties to surface. This is because meditation enables the mind to abandon its normal coping mechanisms and powers of denial. This is most likely to occur in patients who have not confronted difficult emotional problems in their lives, and meditation must be used with caution by such people. It is not usually recommended for people with epilepsy or organic psychiatric problems, including manic depression and schizophrenia.

How can I find a teacher?

There are numerous TM centres across the country, as well as a number of Buddhist centres, where meditation is taught. The FWBO teaches from centres concentrated in London, but their courses are also available in other parts of England and in Scotland. The School of Meditation is based in London and offers introductory talks as well as individual sessions.

How much will it cost?

A few fortunate individuals can obtain transcendental meditation on the NHS if their GPs are fervent believers and are also in fund-holding practices. Otherwise, courses will generally set you back several hundred pounds, although Buddhist meditation is available for much less, around £50 for a six-week course involving at least one session a day. Other organizations, including the School of Meditation, will agree to different terms of payment based on a sliding scale according to your income.

The sceptic's view

The sceptic finds it difficult to take the image of any sensible person sitting cross-legged with arms resting on thighs and index fingers touching thumbs at all seriously. This is for hippies and shadowy figures of the drug culture who don't have enough to do in life. The changes in brain-wave activity and muscle and skin tone are much less dramatic than those induced by formal exercise, which also boasts many of the benefits claimed by followers of meditation. Who, these days, has got 20 minutes twice a day to devote to sitting on one's rear end thinking of nothing at all? Descartes may have said 'I think therefore I am', but the sceptic says, 'I know I am so I don't need to think.'

The therapist's view

'I have been teaching meditation for over 10 years and find that its popularity and acceptance have increased dramatically during that time. In terms of the complete relaxation and inner peace which it can bring about, there are few alternatives that come anywhere near to approaching its simple efficacy and beauty. A proportion of the people I see for the first time are slightly suspicious and sceptical about what it might achieve. Within a matter of days, however, they are grateful for the new calmness and mental control in their lives which they soon discover. Patients' report a better quality of sleep, a reduction in irritability and tension, and even an enhanced creativity, concentration and intelligence. I encourage them to practise transcendental meditation using their mantra at least twice a day which I unfailingly carry out myself. This has given me an inner strength and emotional resolve I could never have achieved in any other way. For many people TM is the rock on which their lives are founded.'

Colin Douglas

The patient's view

'Like many of my medical colleagues, I sometimes used to dread getting up in

the morning and facing another hectic day's work. So much responsibility, so many demands, so little time for myself. I started to use transcendental meditation after an exhilarating hiking trek in the Himalayas and found its incredible ability to relax me worked just as well back home. I now meditate for 20 minutes morning and evening on a daily basis and this enables me to face the world with a calmness I never believed possible. I never feel stressed now, and actually believe I have become more creative and effective as a result of this wonderful mental exercise.'

David Whitton

Naturopathy

Origins

Amongst other things, Hippocrates recommended special diets, fasting, exercise, hydrotherapy and manipulative therapy for his patients, and can therefore certainly be regarded as the father of naturopathic medicine. The ancient Greeks were known to have built healing temples adjacent to thermal springs, and these have also attracted well-to-do Europeans over the last two centuries. The natural spa waters of Bath and Tunbridge Wells and the mineral salts of Epsom are just as famous in Britain as Vichy is in France or Baden Baden in Germany.

Early in the twentieth century, well-known naturopaths, like Stanley Lief and Alfred Vogel, established residential nature cure resorts offering natural and holistic therapy embracing a number of different disciplines. Essential to them all were hydrotherapy, therapeutic fasting, healthy eating, colonic irrigation, detoxification, osteopathy and psychotherapy. Falling out of favour somewhat in the 1950s and 1960s due to widespread over-confidence in modem scientific technology and potent pharmaceutical drugs, naturopathy then enjoyed a resurgence of popularity when the limitations and side effects of modern medicine came to be more widely realized. Naturopathy today remains very popular and several aspects of it are recognized and practised by many orthodox NHS doctors.

What is naturopathy?

Naturopathy is a therapeutic system based on the belief that the body has the power to heal itself through its own inner vitality. Given the right set of natural resources, it can achieve maximal health and prevent the onset of disease. Not only do naturopaths maintain this idea of the body's vital force, but they see illness as evidence that the body is not in harmony and perfect balance with the environment around it, and that a patient's symptoms are a sign that the natural healing processes of the body are at work. As such, symptoms of illness are regarded by the naturopath as welcome indicators that the body is actively fighting off illness, and should not therefore be repressed. One controversial aspect of the naturopathic philosophy is that childhood illnesses, such as measles and mumps, play an important part in stimulating the immune system and rendering it capable of fighting more important diseases in the future, like rheumatism or even cancer. Naturopaths therefore recommend that children are not vaccinated but are nursed through any illness using natural remedies. Indeed, they are loath to treat symptoms of even the mildest infections, such as diarrhoea or colds and coughs, since the symptoms, which are so unpleasant to the patient, are in fact the body's most natural way of eradicating any germs or toxins.

All naturopathic treatment is natural and is designed to support the body's inborn healing ability and innate homeostatic mechanisms. To achieve this, clean water, whole foods, fresh air and exercise, sunlight and relaxation may all be prescribed. The naturopath aims to balance the body's physical structure, its emotions and its biochemistry in a 'triad' of health, so whilst osteopathy helps to correct musculo-skeletal malalignments, fasting and diet are used to stimulate biochemical homeostasis, and psychotherapy is used to abolish unresolved emotions which can be disruptive to the hormonal or digestive systems. Another basic tenet of naturopathy is the 'law of cure' which basically maintains that patients with chronic diseases undergoing a naturopathic treatment may experience an exacerbation of their symptoms prior to feeling better. This is seen as evidence of the underlying cause of the symptoms coming to the surface, and as a tangible demonstration that it is being eradicated.

How does it work?

Naturopathy is supposed to work by making adjustments to the body's internal environment so that its own vital curative force can bring about healing. The treatment is varied and very much tailored to the individual. The following components are considered important:

Diet

This is probably the most important aspect in naturopathy and is designed to strengthen the body where necessary or free it from toxins or allergens if appropriate. Most naturopathic diets concentrate on whole foods and vegetarian organic foods, which are eaten in their raw state to retain the vitamins and minerals which would otherwise be reduced through cooking. Elimination diets may be incorporated into the patient's treatment if allergies or intolerances are suspected. Fasting or basic whole food diets are therefore commonly prescribed for any patient attending a naturopathic clinic.

Fasting

In order to detoxify the body, patients may be advised to go on a complete or partial fast for up to seven days at a time. Even fit, healthy people are recommended at least one day's fast each month. Two well-known types of fast are the grape fast, on which the patient eats up to 2.75 kg (6 lb) grapes each day, and drinks only water, and the Guelpa saline fast, a three-day salt-water fast for people with rheumatic disorders.

Osteopathy

In the belief that spinal structure affects bodily functions elsewhere, the naturopath will also employ manipulative techniques as part of their therapy. Gentle soft tissue techniques, such as neuro-muscular technique (NMT), are often used for this purpose for the elderly and the chronically ill.

Hydrotherapy

Central to naturopathic practice, this is employed to stimulate circulation, to enhance vitality or to relieve pain and discomfort. Cold water may be used to invigorate and tone, hot water is used to relax, and sometimes alternate hot and cold water bathing may be used to encourage lymphatic drainage and blood flow around the body, and to reduce inflammation or bruising in areas of strain, stress or disease. Sitz baths involve the patient sitting alternately in hot and cold water, and are helpful for people with problems in the lower abdominal or pelvic areas, such as period problems, diverticulitis or constipation.

Psychotherapy

Since, in the triad of health, naturopaths regard a patient's psychological state as central to their overall condition, practitioners attempt to remove negative thoughts and destructive emotions which hold the patient back from achieving their full potential. Counselling and relaxation techniques are often used for this purpose, and the patient is encouraged and supported throughout.

Other techniques

These include many of the complementary therapies described elsewhere in this book, including herbalism, homeopathy, iridology, radionics, or even crystal therapy.

Is naturopathy effective?

The idea that we are all surrounded by harmful by-products of twentieth-century living is a very popular one. Most people in Britain would agree that we eat far too many processed, chemically altered foods, and too much saturated fat, and consume too much alcohol. Pollution surrounds us in terms of cigarette smoke, industrial pollution, petrol fumes and atmospheric contamination. Even without knowing it, our intake of the pesticides and insecticides used in farming, and of the additives and preservatives used in mass-produced foods, is quite considerable, so anything natural we can do to counteract any potentially harmful effects is sure to be welcome. The importance of antioxidants in mopping up free radicals (see page 259) may well have been underappreciated in the past and may well account for our high rate of coronary heart disease and cancer. If so, many of the basic tenets of naturopathy are well founded.

Scientific evidence suggests that special diets for sufferers of rheumatoid arthritis may well improve their symptoms. A year-long study in 1991 suggested that their grip strength, their pain levels and the inflammation of their joints all improved when put on a specifically chosen diet following a period of fasting. Another study published in the *Journal of Clinical Rheumatology* in the same year supported the results. These findings should be carefully scrutinized, however. Few Consultant Rheumatologists working within the NHS and who see patients crippled with the most severe forms of inflammatory arthritis would agree that the diseases can be significantly altered by dietary manipulation. In fact, some have pointed out that elimination diets can be positively harmful in that they are restrictive and can make an already poorly and depressed patient even more miserable. Naturopaths, on the other hand, disagree, but do acknowledge that any dietary change should be carried out gradually, particularly for frail patients whose quality of life is already reduced. They also acknowledge the likelihood of a 'crisis of healing' when the patient's symptoms get worse before they get better, a fact that they are always at pains to explain to the patient before treatment commences.

What form might the treatment take?

The patient's first session with a naturopath will be similar to one with an ordinary doctor. A full medical history will be taken, and a full physical examination carried out, as well as occupational and family details being documented. Diagnostic tests may be used, including the more controversial ones such as iridology, hair or nail analysis and radionics. Next, the patient will be given some kind of dietary diary to keep for several weeks, and, based on this, dietary changes will subsequently be suggested. The recommended diet usually includes a lot of organic fruit and vegetables, the elimination of sugar and other refined carbohydrates and very little protein, all of which should preferably be of plant origin. Abstinence from or a severe reduction in alcohol, coffee and tea intake is also generally recommended. Smoking, needless to say, is strongly discouraged. Complete fasting, or juice fasting for the beginner, may be proposed, and hydrotherapy of one kind or another will form part of the new regime. Naturopaths do not encourage the use of medicines for symptom relief as they see symptoms merely as evidence of the body trying to heal itself, and are therefore hostile to the idea of routine antibiotic prescription.

What problems are helped by naturopathy?

Being a holistic therapy in the true sense, naturopaths believe that patients' wellbeing and overall good health can be enhanced by the adoption of its practices. Naturopathy therefore claims to be able to help anyone with almost any condition, although it should not encourage patients to think they are ever totally cured. Many chronic conditions for which orthodox medicine is inadequate, such as ME (myalgic encephalomyelitis) and rheumatoid arthritis, may be improved, and sufferers of irritable bowel syndrome, recurrent migraine and intractable eczema may benefit. Premenstrual syndrome, sinus problems, asthma and hay fever, food intolerances and allergies and constipation, are all conditions which may show significant response in the hands of the naturopath. Furthermore, the osteopathic soft tissue techniques used can help many with musculo-skeletal disorders, and this includes children as well as the frail and elderly. Many people are led to believe that naturopaths can boost the immune system, in order to prevent illness from occurring in the future, but what 'boosting the immune system' actually means, and whether this is scientifically true remains to be seen.

Is it safe?

Not all things which are natural are safe and without risk, but in the hands of a qualified practitioner naturopathy is safe for all. All age groups can benefit, ranging from the very young through to the pregnant woman and the elderly.

How can I find a naturopath ?

To ensure that the naturopath is fully trained, find one who is registered with the General Council and Register of Naturopaths. Their members sport the letters MRN after their name, are covered by full indemnity insurance and are bound by a recognized code of conduct and ethics. Many will have trained at the British College of Naturopathy and Osteopathy in London. Failure to select a therapist who is a member of the General Council exposes any patient to the risk of being treated by an unskilled and unsafe naturopath.

How much will it cost?

Patients can expect to pay up to £50 for the first consultation and about half as much for subsequent sessions. If you are happy with the treatment, you may wish to continue seeing your naturopath, and many people with ongoing problems make a visit once every few weeks.

The sceptic's view

The sceptic regards the naturopath with some suspicion. An orthodox physician abhors any advice which discourages parents from vaccinating their children as it exposes them once again to the appalling complications of otherwise minor childhood diseases such as mumps, measles and meningitis. Encephalitis, which caused so much devastation and high perinatal mortality at the turn of the century, is an example. The idea that symptoms should not be treated and are merely evidence that the body's inner healing powers are fighting disease is abhorrent to the conventionally trained doctor who would also point out that the naturopath's disdain for antibiotics would result in hundreds of thousands of our population dying from septicaemia, meningitis and endocarditis if naturopaths were free to practise unopposed. Naturopaths can reasonably allow patients to play with water, have their tummies massaged and their food improved, but they certainly shouldn't put people on strict elimination diets for no reason, withhold life-saving therapies and examine samples of their nail clippings in the forlorn hope of diagnosing some internal illness. By all means, patients should enjoy all things natural in life, especially fresh air, sunlight and relaxation, but the sceptic still holds the view that they shouldn't need to pay £50 for the privilege.

The therapist's view

'As a naturopathic physician, every patient who comes to me is a new challenge, because together we must embark on a journey of exploration into his or her potential for health.

'Unlike the other major complementary medicine disciplines, naturopathy is not based on a particular type of treatment but is an approach to health which recognizes that the body has an inherent vitality striving to keep us in balance and feeling well. Our job is to involve the patient in discovering what may have interfered with the smooth running of that process and in attempting to correct it with natural, non-toxic measures.

'It is encouraging to see the benefits of many of the traditional naturopathic recommendations in nutrition and dietary therapy being confirmed by the latest research in nutritional biochemistry. For example, naturopaths have always advocated fresh raw vegetables and fruit, and whole grain produce as an essential part of a basic healthy diet.

'But there is much more to naturopathy than prescribing diets and supplements. Hydrotherapy to relieve pain, stimulate the immune system or simply to help sleep; special soft tissue techniques in osteopathic treatment; and stress management all contribute to the integrated approach upon which we base our practice.

'Thanks to research, we also have new ways of testing for disturbances of function in the body under everyday conditions which enable us to be more precise in advising our patients on how to help themselves.

'Naturopathy provides a safe and effective approach to a wide range of disorders, including childhood diseases, skin problems, respiratory troubles, such as sinusitis, bronchitis, and asthma, and digestive disorders. Perhaps more rewarding is the possibility of providing a practical approach to the diagnosis and treatment of the growing catalogue of vague symptoms which do not fit any particular disease category.

'As a principal participant in the emerging field of functional medicine, naturopathy continues to emphasize treatment of the patient rather than the disease. And each patient has a unique capacity for response.'

R. Newman Turner, BAc, ND, DO, MRN, FBAcC

The patient's view

'I first went to see a naturopath because my complexion was awful, I was suffering from a condition called candida, which my family doctor failed to recognize, and because I had symptoms suggestive of sinusitis. I did not feel I was getting effective or sympathetic treatment from my doctor so I tried naturopathy. Within a week or two I soon realized I was going to have to look at the whole of the way I lived my life. I was given a detailed diet which included fasting, I had long sessions talking over the way I felt about my life in general, I had manipulation on my spine and other joints and also enjoyed hydrotherapy and iridology diagnosis. I feel so much better than I used to and I'm a great believer in juicing, which I still use regularly in addition to fasting. Whenever I'm feeling a little down, I go back to my naturopath for a therapeutic boost.'

Sandy Brice

Nutritional Therapy

Origins

On a very primitive level the origins of nutritional therapy were simple: if Neanderthal man did not eat, he died. The whole *raison d'être* of our earliest ancestors was to find enough sustenance to prevent them starving and to keep them alive. Later, as animal husbandry and agriculture developed the concept of using particular foodstuffs and herbs as remedies for certain medical conditions became popular. Regrettably, it remained a spectacularly hit-and-miss affair for centuries. Even as recently as 250 years ago, sailors were suffering from the terrible effects of scurvy purely because no one had noticed that protracted deficiency of vitamin C in the diet made their gums bleed and their teeth fall out. Deficiencies of other vitamins are known to cause all sorts of other symptoms, ranging from anaemia and night blindness right through to skin diseases and nerve damage. It was not until the middle of the twentieth century that the vital importance of all the food components in our diet was first appreciated. Those components broadly consist of protein, carbohydrate, fat and a large number of vitamins and minerals.

Clinical nutrition, which is the dietary advice handed out by orthodox doctors to patients suffering with recognized and defined conditions, is based on this. A patient with irritable bowel syndrome, for example, would be recommended a higher fibre intake, someone with anaemia more red meat and spinach, and a diabetic a sugar-free diet, and so on. A new development in the 1960s introduced for the first time the notion of sub-clinical deficiencies, which hypothesized that sub-optimal vitamin and mineral intakes could result in a wide-ranging spectrum of symptoms. Deficiencies sometimes too subtle to be scientifically measurable were proposed as the underlying problem. This far from obvious form of malnutrition was never likely to be sufficient to produce gross evidence of disease, such as the anaemia seen in iron deficiency or the bowed limbs of rickets caused by vitamin D deficiency, but was nevertheless capable of leading to nebulous, non-specific and very common complaints like fatigue, lethargy, generalized aches and pains and susceptibility to common infections.

The idea was first put forward in the USA by Professor Linus Pauling who coined such tongue-twisting phrases as orthomolecular psychiatry and orthomolecular medicine which described the theory that the mind and body could only function to their maximum potential in the best possible molecular environment. More recently, biomedical research has concentrated very specifically on the importance of antioxidant components within the diet. These are naturally occurring molecules capable of disarming potentially harmful by-products of metabolism called free radicals, which otherwise accumulate in the body as a result of smoking, environmental pollution, radiation, or eating a fatty diet, and which may accelerate or trigger a host of serious diseases. Amongst the growing list of ailments strongly linked to antioxidant deficiency are cancer, arthritis, cataracts, senile dementia, heart attack, stroke and diabetes. Some scientists also now believe sub-optimal antioxidant components in the diet can even contribute to infertility, macular degeneration (retinal deterioration at the back of the eye causing blindness), mental illness and periodontal disease.

What is nutritional therapy?

Basically, nutritional therapy entails using foods to prevent and treat ill-health. On a simple level, it might mean suggesting to someone who is constipated that they eat more fibre such as bran-based cereals and fresh fruit and vegetables. It might also mean advising a patient with coronary heart disease to eat less saturated fat by changing to leaner cuts of red meat and low-fat dairy products. On another level, however, nutritional therapy would attempt to prevent the many illnesses listed above which an inadequate or sub-optimal diet might engender.

Practitioners of nutritional therapy regard many people in today's modern world as being overfed but undernourished – rendered obese by the empty calories in the food served by our fast food restaurants, yet nutritionally impoverished by the lack of overall goodness and purity of what we eat. Nutritional therapy attempts to correct this imbalance by advising clients about a more appropriate and healthy diet. This would involve a dietary regime, designed not only to keep them healthier in the future but also to treat any symptoms existing at the current time. Some therapists would even provide recommendations about food to remedy particular medical complaints such as persistent catarrh and mucus production, digestive problems, premenstrual problems, asthma, eczema and rheumatism.

Nutritional therapy also addresses the fashionable but nevertheless highly significant matter of food intolerance and food allergy. It sets about identifying those foods in our diet which may produce problems, and then eradicating them from our menus. It remains a highly controversial medical area in many aspects, but even where concrete and incontrovertible evidence has proved the benefits of dietary adjustment in particular areas, conventionally trained doctors have still appeared rather slow on the uptake. Complementary practitioners working in the field of nutritional therapy, on the other hand, are highly aware of the esoteric and subtle manifestations of food intolerance, and can assist patients accordingly in an attempt to eradicate their symptoms.

Generally speaking, nutritional therapists are also proponents of the concept of 'toxic overload'. These toxins, supposedly derived from environmental or self-induced pollution, include amongst other things pesticides, preservatives, food colourings, additives, hormones, nicotine and alcohol. Radioactivity, sunlight, drugs and stress all contribute as does a high-fat diet. This dissolves these pollutants more easily and is therefore capable of introducing them into the body in highly concentrated forms. Toxins are also produced within our bodies as a normal by-product of metabolism by the action of intestinal bacteria on food residues. Nutritional practitioners seek to flush out and eradicate these toxins by the careful avoidance or selection of specific foodstuffs. Where appropriate this may include a recommendation to switch to organically produced food.

How does it work?

There is broad agreement now on what constitutes a healthy diet, as outlined by the WHO and government guidelines. It is a varied menu which incorporates all the essential components, mainly protein, carbohydrate, fat, minerals and vitamins, and all in the correct proportion. A healthy diet should be low in fat, high in fibre, with no more than 30 per cent of our total calorie intake coming from fat and no more than 30 per cent of that consisting of the saturated variety. A minimum of five pieces of fresh fruit or vegetables should be consumed each day. Our diet should be tailored to suit our individual needs and lifestyles, and then adjusted to our state of health or lack of it. Nutritional therapy goes further than this, however, as it does not recognize that existing recommended allowances (RDAs) of vitamins and minerals are sufficient, and believes that millions of people suffer symptoms unduly as a result of sub-optimal nutrition. Antioxidant supplementation is considered vital, and the following is a brief explanation of how it is supposed to work.

Oxygen is the life-giving element in all plant and animal life. Without it, the cells in our bodies cannot metabolize food at all, and it controls every biological process in our bodies. However, oxygen is also chemically reactive and can oxidize neighbouring molecules just like it oxidizes the paint scratches on a car, causing rust. These oxidized molecules are known as free radicals and wander aimlessly around the body like microscopic lager louts looking for trouble wherever they can find it. Moreover, free radicals are an especial menace because the cellular damage caused by their oxidation process gradually leads to serious diseases (like cancer, arthritis and hardening of the arteries. Antioxidants are our saviours. These are the 'goody' chemicals that neutralize and eradicate free radicals. They are prevalent in many naturally occurring foods, but particularly good sources are the vitamins A, C and E, betacarotene and the mineral selenium. Other lesser known sources, such as bioflavonoids and pycnogenols, are becoming increasingly recognized, but there are hundreds of others present in commonly consumed food. The balance between the antioxidants in someone's diet and their exposure to free radicals may ultimately represent the balance between life and death. Nutritional therapists try to tip this balance in the patient's favour by weighting the scales more heavily against the molecular nasties lurking in their body, which may be regularly reinforced by poor and inappropriate eating habits.

Common culprits responsible for true food allergies include dairy products, wheat, flour, nuts, eggs, shellfish, citrus fruits and yeast. In susceptible people, these may result in skin rashes, diarrhoea and vomiting, abdominal cramps and bloating, and sometimes swelling of the lips and tongue and breathing difficulties. In the case of the increasingly common peanut allergy, these symptoms can be even more dramatic, producing acute clinical shock with breathing difficulties and collapse, known as angioneurotic oedema, which can rapidly become life-threatening unless urgently treated. Food intolerance, on the other hand, is much less dramatic in the way it manifests itself, and can appear in a vast array of different guises. Intolerance to food colourings and preservatives, for example, can bring about attention deficit hyperactivity disorder (ADHD) and behavioural problems in children, whereas reactions to citrus fruit, cereal protein or lactose sugars in cow's milk can lead to unexplained bloating and abdominal pains in adults. If such an intolerance or allergy is suspected, a nutritional therapist might well start his patient on an exclusion or elimination diet designed specifically to identify the offending foodstuffs. This needs expert supervision, however, as exclusion diets are never easy to follow and can deprive patients of essential nutrients unless supplementation is considered.

Is nutritional therapy effective?

Orthodox physicians have long practised basic forms of nutritional therapy. Recommending calcium-rich milk for brittle bones, iron-packed lean red meat for anaemia and vitamin C-laden citrus fruits to prevent colds, are examples. They have often correctly advised patients with gout to avoid fortified wines, whilst recommending a judicious glass or two of good claret each day to patients eager to reduce their risk of heart disease. The benefits of a high-fibre diet, particularly when based on a high intake of fresh fruit and vegetable, are irrefutable. In developing countries, the incidence of colon cancer is totally insignificant compared to ours because high-residue foods are eaten as a staple part of the diet, and because much less saturated fat is consumed. Moreover, all the non-malignant intestinal disease, like diverticulitis, irritable bowel syndrome and haemorrhoids, occur much less frequently too. However, the real question is this: can the nutritional therapist achieve even greater results in terms of promoting good health and preventing illness than conventional doctors? According to a growing body of clinical researchers, they almost certainly can.

The work of Professor Diplock at Guy's Hospital in London suggests that it is increasingly likely that the role of antioxidants has indeed been greatly underestimated in terms of serious disease prevention in the past. One such antioxidant is vitamin E and a huge clinical study on this conducted on 87,000 or more nurses in 1993, and published in the *New England Journal of Medicine* showed that taking supplements of this vitamin significantly reduced the risks of heart disease as opposed to not taking enough vitamin E, which increased the risks. Other studies have shown that disorders notoriously immune to the ministrations of conventional doctors such as migraine, multiple sclerosis, premenstrual syndrome, irritable bowel syndrome, ME (myalgic encephalomyelitis) and certain skin problems may all respond encouragingly, if not at times dramatically to nutritional therapy. Many patients, particularly women, in whom the hormonal element may play a role, have been amazed to witness how even minor adjustments in their dietary regime can result in freedom from abdominal bloating, fluid retention and chronic fatigue even after years of suffering. A small but significant number of parents have also reported amazingly positive behavioural changes in their children with hyperactivity or attention deficit disorder after relatively painless elimination of food additives from their diets. Since the antioxidant revolution is still relatively new, but gaining ground, it remains to be seen whether there really will be less cancer, arthritis and heart disease in the future, and whether people will live longer and age more gracefully. However, since these substances are extremely safe, even in overdosage, these seem compelling reasons for turning to a nutritional intake richer in a variety of fresh fruit and vegetables, and a diet less dominated by large quantities of saturated fat.

What form might the treatment take?

Nutritional therapists may be conventionally qualified doctors or practitioners of other complementary therapies such as homeopathy, traditional Chinese or Western herbalism or naturopathy. The typical consultation incorporates taking a full history and documenting the person's lifestyle, smoking and drinking habits, physical activities and work and social relationships. Any medication taken, such as antibiotics or the contraceptive pill, are of particular interest. Some therapists will ask for a questionnaire to be filled in or request samples of blood, urine, sweat or hair for testing. Any current symptoms are taken into account and special care is taken to evaluate any possible food intolerance or allergy or exposure to environmental toxins. After due consideration based on an analysis of this data, the practitioner will then usually draw up a dietary regime tailored to the individual patient, and suggest any vitamin, mineral or herbal supplementation required.

What problems are helped by nutritional therapy?

Since up to a third of all cancers are attributed to poor diet, and since too much fat in our typical Western cuisine accounts for the excessively high mortality from heart disease and strokes in the UK, a healthy diet is obviously highly advisable for every single one of us. Applied nutritional therapy can offer some patients the chance to enhance their energy levels and abolish any long-standing and irritating symptoms they may be experiencing as a result of food intolerance or toxic overload. Migraine sufferers may benefit from the avoidance of trigger factors such as Chianti and other red wines, cheese and chocolate. Those troubled by premenstrual syndrome can benefit from essential fatty acids, gammalinolenic acid (GLA), oil of evening primrose, pyridoxine, vitamin B_6, and magnesium supplements. Other ailments which respond to dietary manipulation include arthritis, high blood pressure (through reduced salt intake), chronic fatigue (including ME), constipation, irritable bowel syndrome and skin disorders such as eczema. Menopausal symptoms, such as hot flushes and night sweats may be significantly reduced; soya milk, for instance, is thought to reduce these by as much as 40 per cent when the sufferer consumes just 500 ml (18 fl oz) a day, either in a drink or as an ingredient of cooking. Conditions such as anxiety and depression, osteoporosis, neuralgia and a tendency to suffer frequent colds and infections may all respond. Pregnant women can also derive considerable benefit from caring about what they eat, both preconceptually and post-natally, as can their unborn babies, whose overall nutritional status is of paramount importance.

Is it safe?

Rigid elimination diets and highly restrictive regimes are generally not safe because they are capable of producing a different or opposite effect to what is intended. However, few nutritional therapists ever attempt this and only the most expert should ever try. In all other respects, nutritional therapy is entirely safe for everyone. The patient's doctor should always be informed about what is intended as the nutritional therapist needs to realize that some supplements may be hazardous in certain individual's situations. When used carefully, however, by experienced, professional practitioners, nutritional therapy is safe for people of all ages, babies and octogenarians alike.

How can I find a nutritional therapist?

Many NHS or private doctors retain a special interest in nutrition and practise as nutritional therapists. Other practitioners work in various fields of complementary therapy. The best-known umbrella organization in the UK is the Society for the Promotion of Nutritional Therapy which maintains a professional register of therapists and can tell you if there is one local to you. The Women's Nutritional Advisory Service also comes highly recommended. However, it is imperative to be wary of the growing number of 'cowboy' organizations springing up which advertise freely and claim to be able to diagnose subtle nutritional deficiencies on the strength of a blood test or hair sample without any scientific evidence to support this. Several have been exposed by investigators who have sent two identical blood samples taken at the same time from the same person, only to be sent back two analyses which are totally and fundamentally different. These analyses are not only expensive, but entirely bogus.

How much will it cost?

The average consultation and treatment session with a registered nutritional therapist will cost about £40, with the cost of any supplements on top. Companies who act alone and often with no accreditation or authority, but who claim to be able to diagnose previously undetected food intolerance or allergy from a blood sample sent through the post may charge upwards of £200. There is a high risk that this is money down the drain.

The sceptic's view

Nutritional therapy does not exist in countries where there is simply not enough to eat. People living there are too busy just trying to survive. The idea that all the millions of people in our civilized society who are grossly overweight are actually undernourished is arrant nonsense. They are stuffed so full of nutrients their bodies simply do not know how to handle them all. If they want to spend money they cannot really afford by taking additional supplements all they end up doing is excreting them. Of course, many of them would do well to eat less fat and more fibre, but then that is fairly obvious and you do not really need a nutritional therapist to tell you that food intolerance is another hugely exaggerated phenomenon. Only about 5 per cent of all so-called hyperactive children have any real food allergy or intolerance to account for it. As for the antioxidant story, to the sceptic it just sounds like a hard commercial sell. Vitamins and minerals available in supplements but which cannot be provided in sufficient amounts in even the healthiest natural foods? And which prevent cancer, arthritis and the ageing process? And stop hardening of the arteries causing heart attacks and stroke? And senile dementia? And what else? Make you look like Claudia Schiffer or Pierce Brosnan? The sceptic is not impressed.

The therapist's view

'It is quite common for overburdened individuals to neglect their own needs, failing to find time to exercise or relax and eating the wrong foods for comfort, or skipping meals altogether. Our diets have changed dramatically over the last 50 years, to the point where many are no longer meeting their basic needs. Repeated research at the Women's Nutritional Advisory Service (WNAS) has shown that women of childbearing age often have nutritional deficiencies, which affect both their brain chemistry and hormone levels, often resulting in unwanted incapacitating symptoms.

'In the 15 years of working with patients at the WNAS, we have been able to help literally thousands of patients over their long-term ills, and to remove unwanted and unjustified 'labels' that they thought they would wear for life. We have dealt with thousands of patients who have previously been labelled psychologically ill, and have left them symptom free after three or four months. Patients who have had severe migraine for years no longer even have headaches; we have former acne sufferers without spots; and irritable bowel victims who no longer have to pay attention to their digestion. The violent, and often suicidal premenstrual syndrome sufferer, who previously described herself as Jekyll and Hyde, feels like her old self again all month; ongoing problems with thrush and cystitis have abated; and the turbulent symptoms of the menopause have, in the majority of cases, been replaced by a new vitality for life. These are just some of the weekly achievements at the WNAS. They are not miracles, just the application of existing medical science relating to diet, exercise, relaxation and nutritional supplements. Being able to help people to feel better than they have felt for years is a very satisfying occupation.'

Maryon Stewart, WNAS

The patient's view

'My problem was premenstrual tension (PMT) and what it meant for me was palpitations, insomnia, an inability to speak properly and lack of co-ordination (I was a liability in my car!). I had terrible rages when I screamed and shouted at everyone. I felt so inadequate and guilty; I hated myself; life was hell! I was always looking for a solution. I tried hormones for seven months but by the end I had breakthrough bleeding and enormous tender breasts.

'So after this latest failure I found the Women's Nutritional Advisory Service, who put me on what they called a resting diet, which consisted of plenty of fresh fruit and vegetables, no gluten (so no wheat, barley, oats and rye), plenty of oily fish and a little meat (white only) plus some vitamin supplements. I didn't know how I could cope without coffee as I was a 10–12-cups-a-day person, but amazingly I did. I came off chocolate, biscuits and sweets, and went on to keep fit three times a week.

'I felt fantastic, and quite quickly, too. No more painful bloating and swollen fingers. I had clear skin for a change and I was sleeping well. My mental capacity improved along with my co-ordination. I had loads of energy and had finally found an answer to my problem, so no more PMT. I could hardly believe such a natural and simple process could change my life so radically. I've changed from being a raging loony into a person who I know is the real me.'

Sue Cleasby

Osteopathy

Origins

Osteopathy was developed in the 1870s by Andrew Taylor Still, an American doctor who had originally trained as an engineer. After working in the army as a surgeon, he became disillusioned with conventional medicine and the brutality and lack of compassion involved in its practices. He also lost three of his own children to meningitis and realized that other methods of treatment beyond the realms of conventional scientific thinking were needed.

Still's engineering instincts told him that for normal function, a sound structure was required, and the fundamental principle that 'structure governs function' remains at the heart of modern-day osteopathy. Still believed that if the human body possessed sound structural integrity, then the body's own self-healing mechanisms would allow normal healthy functions to continue. It was Still who called this form of treatment 'osteopathy' derived from the Greek words *osteo* (bone) and *pathos* (disease). He believed that the spine was the most important part of the body, not only because it surrounds and protects the sensitive spinal cord, but also because it houses that part of the nervous system which governs each and every area of the body, controlling all our senses and directing every single movement and both conscious and unconscious thought. He believed that misalignment of bones, ligaments and joints in this area, and tensions in the muscles surrounding them, was capable of having a widespread effect on every other organ in the body. By applying manipulative techniques to these problems, he came to believe that physical and emotional problems could be remedied. The theory was reinforced when his patients seemed to fare a great deal better than those having conventional therapy.

Still set up his first school of osteopathic medicine in 1892 in Kirksville, Missouri, and one of his students set up England's first college, the British School of Osteopathy, in 1917. Now, over 5 million people every year see an osteopath and, following the Osteopathy Act of 1993, it became the very first complementary therapy to be regulated by law, and therefore totally recognized by the orthodox medical fraternity.

What is osteopathy?

Broadly speaking, osteopathy involves physical manipulation of the body's musculo-skeletal system – the bones, ligaments, joints and muscles – in order to diagnose problems and to alleviate pain, enhance mobility and improve general health. Based on the belief that structure governs function, the manipulative techniques are employed to influence not just the parts of the musculo-skeletal system being realigned and physically altered, but to improve function in peripheral and distant organs as well.

For example, pins and needles in the hand caused by irritation of nerves from a misaligned joint in the neck can be abolished through osteopathy. But since osteopathy has an effect on the nervous system, and since this is linked to every muscle, organ and gland in the body, osteopaths also believe that abdominal organs, the heart and lungs, the skin and the hormonal system can all be positively influenced by its use.

How does it work?

A number of manipulative techniques are used to correct a patient's problems. The techniques used are standard and well established, ranging from simple massage to relax tense muscles, stretching, to improve joint mobility, and high velocity thrust techniques which although more forceful and vigorous than others, should not be violent or painful. Cranial osteopathy employs an even lighter touch and may be used on children and the elderly (see page 180).

Soft tissue manipulation

In soft tissue manipulation, the aim is to encourage tense muscles to relax, fluid retention to drain away through lymphatic channels and flaccid, floppy muscles to tone up.

Neuro-muscular techniques (NMT)

These involve the osteopath using his or her thumb to probe for 'knots' or focal points of soft tissue tension. Fibrositis or scar tissue deep within a muscle can be alleviated in this way.

Articulatory techniques

Articulatory techniques involve the passive movement of joints, the osteopath moving the articulatory surfaces of the joint without the patient helping. A limb, either an arm or leg is used as a lever to put the joints through a full range of movement and a bit beyond. Adhesions, which are strands of tissue binding joints or muscles together abnormally, can be broken down using these techniques, and ligaments and tendons can be stretched. Tight structures can therefore be lengthened in this way and people with osteoarthritis of the hip, for example, can benefit. Contracted and fixed ligaments around the spinal joints can be gently stretched using articulatory techniques, and traction (pulling) can be used to stretch a tightened capsule around a joint such as in the shoulder for people suffering from frozen shoulder or chronic back pain with stiffness.

High velocity thrust technique

The high velocity thrust technique, which is used by chiropractors as well as osteopaths, can sometimes bring about dramatic improvements in the range of spinal movement and the relief of pain. The thrust itself is a short-amplitude, sudden movement delivered in a fraction of a second. The osteopath's hands may be used to thrust in opposite directions, which maximizes the force imposed on the joint in question. The joint is first taken to the maximum of its range of movement, and the high velocity thrust then stretches it a little further to free it completely. A noticeable crack or snap is often heard which may sound alarming, but merely represents the popping of tiny gas bubbles in the synovial fluid which normally exists between the joints.

Other techniques

These include 'muscle energy' and indirect techniques, which are generally restricted to sports injury clinics or cranial osteopathy clinics respectively. Visceral osteopathy and naturopathic osteopathy tend to be practised by special-interest therapists, the former diagnosing and treating people with disorders of the abdominal, thoracic and reproductive systems through manipulation of the abdomen or the nerve centres along the spine. The naturopaths use osteopathy as just one aspect of their treatment repertoire to bring about complete overall healing. All osteopaths aim to restore full function through manipulation of the body's organs.

Is osteopathy effective?

There can be no doubt whatsoever that for acute discomfort occurring in otherwise fit healthy adults who spend a lot of time sitting at their desks at the office, osteopathy can bring about dramatic relief of discomfort or pain. Spinal manipulation is also very useful for acute low back pain, and a report recently published by the Royal College of General Practitioners entitled 'Clinical Guidelines for the Management of Acute Low Back Pain' endorsed and recommended the use of manipulative techniques for back pain, especially if that back pain were short-lived and acute. Many scientific studies have shown that spinal manipulation has proved more effective in the treatment of low back pain than exercise or drug therapy. Other studies have shown that low back pain associated with period pain and undiagnosed non-specific back pain also respond better to osteopathic treatment than to other comparable therapies. Osteopathy is not only recognized scientifically by the orthodox medical establishment, but its use is often recommended for patients by the majority of NHS GPs. GP fundholders may remain able to purchase the services of osteopaths on behalf of their NHS patients, but others can certainly recommend good local osteopaths privately.

What form might the treatment take?

At the first consultation the osteopath will ask the patient about their medical history, in particular their current problems, but also enquire about their general lifestyle, their level of physical activity, their occupation and existing symptoms. If any pain or discomfort is present, a detailed enquiry into the nature of this will follow.

Next, an examination will determine the patient's posture and degree of mobility. The physical examination is very detailed and the patient will need to undress for this to be carried out properly. Sometimes X-rays and other diagnostic tests are appropriate. If the patient has any need for urgent pain relief this may be attempted during the first consultation, but generally a treatment plan is drawn up with the second session in mind for the first application of manipulative treatment. Any of the different techniques may be used at this time, and of course the patient is advised about remedial exercises to achieve rehabilitation. Sessions last between 30 minutes and an hour, and since registered osteopaths are rigorously trained, they will refer patients back to the GP if any type of serious pathology, for example malignancy or inflammatory arthritis, is suspected or found.

Many people are confused as to the difference between osteopathy and chiropractic treatment. There are a number of differences: osteopaths work on all areas of the body, whereas chiropractors tend to concentrate on the spine; osteopaths rarely use X-rays, whereas chiropractors often call upon them; osteopaths use soft tissue techniques to a greater degree than chiropractors.

Manipulative therapy is also carried out by physiotherapists, whose work is available free of charge on the NHS. Referrals to osteopaths are more likely these days, now that GP fund-holders are able to divert funds for this purpose on the patient's behalf; but regrettably this is still not yet commonplace.

What problems are helped by osteopathy?

Osteopathy is particularly good at relieving back problems, notably discomfort and limited movement in the neck, and can even relieve pins and needles going down the arm which originate from minor nerve irritation in the cervical spine. Low back pain may also respond well, whether the cause is muscular, ligamentous or articular (coming from the joint). In the same way that neuralgia in the arms can be improved, so can sciatica. Osteopaths also treat sports injuries, migraine and tension headaches, dizziness and giddiness. Many forms of arthritis can be helped, particularly osteoarthritis, and some osteopaths also treat conditions not usually associated with manipulative therapy, such as premenstrual syndrome, asthma and respiratory problems and non-specific abdominal pain and constipation.

Even pregnant women, who are often told by conventionally minded doctors that nothing can be done for their postural backache, may be helped by osteopathy, and after the first three months gentle manipulation here is quite safe. On the face of it, it may be difficult to understand how people with chronic bronchitis and asthma can be helped in this way, but osteopaths argue that since the muscles of the ribcage and diaphragm can be made to relax or tighten in the same way that other muscles can, the depth and quality of breathing can be improved.

Is it safe?

Osteopathy is unlikely to be entirely safe unless you see a fully qualified registered practitioner, but of all the various techniques used, one can usually be found which will be suitable for people of any age and with most conditions. Manipulative therapies are not suitable in certain circumstances, however, particularly in people with brittle bone disease (osteoporosis), women in the first three months of pregnancy, people with rheumatoid arthritis where the joints are actively inflamed, and people with serious nerve entrapment or any disease of the spinal cord itself. Osteopathy should also be avoided if there has been a recent fracture or a whiplash injury in the neck area. Another rarer type of chronic inflammation in the lower part of the back, called ankylosing spondylitis, is also to be avoided by osteopaths. Lastly, any kind of progressive disease process in the bones themselves are a contraindication to osteopathy, so any form of bone cancer, including the blood disorders leukaemia, lymphoma and multiple myeloma, would not be at all suitable for this kind of treatment. Reputable practitioners recognize, of course, these limitations and would appropriately refer patients back to their GP for more suitable treatment. It must be remembered that there are some 5 million consultations every year and the number of reported adverse reactions is very low.

There have been a very small number of deaths from spinal manipulation over the years, and the occasional stroke has been attributed to this treatment. However, more common side effects are nerve compression brought about by the mechanical movement of joints, and the occasional exacerbation of the pain which brought the patient to the practitioner in the first place. Overall, however, osteopathy affords quick and broadly speaking very safe alleviation of discomfort and decreased mobility, and probably has a much safer profile than that of orthodox treatment which involves surgery or potent medication.

How can I find an osteopath?

At the present time, the commonest way of finding an osteopath either involves your own NHS GP recommending someone local whom he or she respects and trusts, or involves the patient taking up a personal recommendation from somebody else, and referring themselves privately. Some GP fund-holders may refer you on the NHS to an osteopath if his budget allows.

It is not a good idea to find an osteopath in the Yellow Pages as they are still at liberty to practise under common law, with a minimum of qualifications, and therefore may not be safe. By 1999 it is hoped that all osteopaths will be registered with the General Osteopathic Council (GOsC) which, once it is established will ensure that all osteopaths are registered and approved. Until then, it is estimated that 5 per cent of osteopaths will work without recognized qualifications. Qualified osteopaths currently use the letters DO (Diploma in Osteopathy) or BSc (OST) after their names. Conventionally trained doctors who have undergone a 13-month full-time post-graduate course at the London College of Osteopathic Medicine use the initials MLCOM after their names. There are, however, five professional bodies to which various practitioners belong, and if an osteopath is registered with any of these, it means they are insured, recognize an established code of ethics and are subject to disciplinary procedures. Until the GOsC is finally established, the best way to find a registered practitioner in your area is to contact the Osteopathic Information Service (OIS).

How much will it cost?

You can expect to pay up to £70 or so in London and other major cities, but it may be as little as £25 in other areas. The first consultation is usually the most expensive and prices tend to fall thereafter. In general, osteopaths would agree that most disorders require a minimum of three treatments, but if, after half a dozen, the symptoms have not improved, an alternative approach should be sought.

The sceptic's view

A critic of osteopathy would question the ability of anybody to realign displaced joints. None of us is entirely symmetrical and most of us have some degree of forwards or sidewards curvature of the spine and minor changes caused by wear and tear in our joints evidenced by X-ray findings. Whilst acknowledging that manipulative techniques can work very well in the hands of physiotherapists who passively or actively move ligaments and bones, the idea that the internal organs, especially those of respiration and digestion, can be altered by manipulation of the spine is somewhat illogical. No alteration in the function or structure of abdominal organs has ever been shown scientifically to result from such mechanical treatments. The sceptic believes that people's spines, hips, necks, shoulders and other joints become stiff because they are not used properly, and are never put through their full range of movements, partly through abuse and neglect, and partly because of the sedentary but stressful lifestyle that most of us lead in today's modern age. Osteopathy is hardly capable of addressing all of these problems in one fell swoop!

The therapist's view

'The body stands a much better chance of functioning well when it is structurally and mechanically sound. When a mechanical fault exists in the spine, local pain and inflammation will ensue. Often this has a knock-on effect, interfering with the blood and nerve supply to various parts of the body, causing numerous symptoms.

'Osteopaths not only introduce treatment, but they also spend time educating their patients on how to prevent further problems, introducing strengthening routines and strengthening exercises, do's and don'ts, and handy hints.

'Osteopathy is both safe and effective. Once proper diagnosis has been established and correct treatment applied by a qualified osteopath there is rarely the possibility of the problem becoming worse. The worst that can happen is nothing, but in the majority of cases there will be an improvement, if not a complete cessation of symptoms.

'If you suffer back pain, you have absolutely nothing to lose in consulting an osteopath. In cases of severe pain, it is advisable to consult your doctor first, to establish the proper course of treatment. As an estimated 80 per cent of back pain is mechanical in origin, osteopathy may well be judged the appropriate form of treatment.'

Garry Trainer, BAc, MRTCM, DO, MBEOA

The patient's view

'I have been suffering from back pain for several years. It seems that every 6 months or so I have an acute flare up of symptoms which used to leave me immobilized and bed-bound for several weeks. I used to control the pain by ingesting large quantities of anti-inflammatory drugs. This worked reasonably well until I unfortunately developed side effects. I then reluctantly had to seek another approach to my problem. It was then that I came across osteopathy for the first time. I had nothing to lose so I gave it a try. It all seemed rather odd to me on my first few treatments, but my recurring back pain was 75 per cent better after just the first treatment, and totally relieved after two more visits. I could not believe it; that something that can be so debilitating could be eased so quickly without the need of medication. I still get the occasional bout of back pain but I can now rest assured that if I do I now have a safe and effective way of treating it.'

Kim Sawyer

Radionics

Origins

Albert Abrams, an American neurologist, believed that diseases were electrical rather than cellular in origin, and that when a patient's body harboured an illness, a different form of body radiation was emitted. This was back in the 1920s when the idea of radiation being universally scattered throughout nature was really somewhat revolutionary. As he worked on his hypothesis, Abrams married the words 'radiation' and 'electronics' together and came up with his principle of radionics.

Initially, Abrams claimed that, when medically examining a patient and percussing (tapping) certain parts of their body he could distinguish between healthy and diseased organs by listening to the quality of the sound that was produced. This in itself was not extraordinary because orthodox doctors do this all the time, but he next claimed that if a healthy person merely held a sample of diseased tissue in their hand he could still detect the exact same changes in sound when he percussed certain organs in their body. Finally, he designed 'Abrams' Black Box', a biodynamometer which he stated was capable of detecting disease in a patient – purely by measuring radiation from a mere drop of blood or lock of hair. He even rented the device out to interested parties for £300 a throw.

The theory that medical diagnosis could be reached through detecting radiation also found favour with students of dowsing or water-divining. Soon 'medical dowsers', or radiesthestists, sprang up, all claiming to be able to take a sample or 'witness' from a patient – such as a lock of hair, nail clipping or an eyelash – and suspend a pendulum over it, observe its oscillation and come up with an accurate diagnosis. The patient did not even have to be present.

What is radionics?

Radionics uses specially designed instruments to analyse and correct energy imbalances which can cause illness and mental, physical or emotional problems. A radionics practitioner will state that he or she can measure someone's energy levels and propose a remedial treatment. The analysis is performed at a distance from the patient, using merely a box of electronic tricks and a 'witness' from the patient.

How does it work?

Radionics is supposed to work by allowing the practitioner to tune into the patient's personal energy field by using the energy field of the 'witness' as a template. The 'witness', a lock of hair for example, will still tell the practitioner what he wants to know about the patient even if they are on the other side of the world, and even if the lock of hair was cut off long ago. By tuning in to the patient's energy field in this way, the practitioner claims he can correct imbalances and restore health.

Is radionics effective?

In 1924, the year of Albert Abrams' death, the Royal Society of Medicine enquired into the efficacy of radionics, and amazingly did not condemn it out of hand. Twelve years later, however, the University of Hanover challenged practitioners of radiesthesia to treat a number of animals. Comparing their findings with those of conventional therapists, the results were frankly alarming. Healthy beasts were diagnosed as being ill, and sick ones as being well, or suffering from a different condition. More recent German research showed in 1992 that there was no evidence that radionics was of any scientific value whatsoever.

What form might the treatment take?

The patient may never see the practitioner, but he or she will certainly need to fill in a detailed case-history. This documents previous medical records, family history, any medications the patient may be taking or has taken, and, of course, any symptoms or difficulties currently being suffered. Enquiries are made into the patient's emotional state, lifestyle and personality. The practitioner will then use this information as well as the the patient's 'witness' to 'tune into' the patient's vibrations. The 'witness' is usually a speck of blood on a piece of blotting paper, a nail clipping or a lock of hair. The practitioner does not 'physically' analyse the 'witness' itself, however, when he or she receives it, so patients should not expect a data sheet or computer read-out about the 'witness' and what it shows.

The 'witness' is merely a connecting link between the practitioner, the black box he or she uses, and the patient. Once a diagnosis is reached, the practitioner will then direct a healing energy via the 'witness' to the patient.

Many radionics practitioners now use an automatic computerized system (ACTS), which can administer any one of thousands of treatments to the patient, via the 'witness', in the appropriate duration and strength.

What problems are helped by radionics?

According to the results of studies carried out by scientists and doctors, the answer to this question is probably 'None', but as Hamlet might argue 'There are more things tween heaven and earth. . . than are dreamt of in [our] philosophy', and there is a case for not allowing alternative therapies to be judged purely by orthodox doctors. Disciples of radionics claim they can improve overall health and well-being in their patients. They believe that allergic conditions such as hay fever and asthma can be cleared up, and that pain, particularly resulting from surgical operations and arthritis, can be alleviated.

Is it safe?

Many conventionally trained doctors are reasonably happy to allow their patients to explore radionics as it can do no physical harm. Others, however, cite cases where paranoia and fear have been induced by the realization that the same powers that enable the 'witness' to be used to heal could theoretically be used to do harm. This would also be beyond the control and knowledge of the patient and, as such, is 'comparable to the frightening effect of voodoo'. Vulnerable people might believe in radionics and black magic, but scientists on the whole do not. The real danger of radionics is that desperate people turn to it instead of to conventional medicine, or even to more acceptable forms of complementary therapy, and risk being totally misdiagnosed and improperly treated.

How can I find a radionics practitioner?

The Radionic Association has its own School of Radionics where pupils can study for up to three years to become fully fledged members and earn the right to use the letters MRadA after their names. A list of practitioners can be obtained from the Radionic Association.

How much will it cost?

The initial analysis of a patient's problems usually costs about £25, and the same amount is charged for subsequent treatments.

The sceptic's view

The sceptic would regard radionics as the epitome of quackery and charlatanism. With no scientific evidence to support it, and practitioners who do not even have to meet their clients to diagnose their ailments, this is absolute nonsense. To receive a piece of dead human tissue, such as a nail clipping or lock of hair, in the post and be able to diagnose a cholesterol gall-stone from it must sound far-fetched to even the most gullible amongst us. And the tissue sample itself is not even analysed! Sometimes the electronic diagnostic box is apparently not even plugged into the electricity supply when it draws its medical conclusions! Truly the work of magic and mysticism! Dr Albert Abrams may have thought quantum physics had something to do with explaining radionics, but Ruth Drown, one of his disciples who carried on his work after his death, took the theories and practice just a little too far. The American Medical Association ridiculed her work and results, and she was ultimately jailed for medical quackery and fraud by the US Food and Drugs Administration.

The therapist's view

'A radionic practitioner's life is very interesting and varied; it can be very demanding but always rewarding. Practitioners mostly work from their own homes and dovetail lifestyle with practice, always being prepared to deal with problems as they arise. Sometimes these completely disrupt the plan for the day.

'Radionic practice is not all healing at a distance. Administration takes time and this has to be done efficiently.

'Most conditions can be helped radionically, if only to help the patient feel better and therefore more able to cope with their symptoms. Conditions vary from, say, a broken ankle, for which healing of bone and tissue is required, to treatment for shock and other psychological disturbances, including stress, which has causes that often emanate from the subtle bodies. Sometimes conditions that seem purely physical have the real cause in the subtle side. About 80 per cent of all humans and about 90 per cent of animals respond to treatment.

'Some patients can be a little trying, but in general they are very grateful and many and varied aspects of life are revealed from all over the world as distance is no object with radionics. It is a very demanding but satisfying way of life, knowing that healing is being directed to human beings and animals, but it must be realized that radionics can be applied to soil and plants as well, which is another vast subject.'

Enid A. Eden

The patient's view

'My mum used to tell me I was always washed out and ill, and was missing too much school with sore throats and runny noses. It is funny because she sent off a little bit of my hair and a drop of blood, which she pricked from my finger on to a piece of blotting paper, to a woman who lives in Cornwall. Some of my friends thought this was weird. My mum says that the last laugh is on them, however, because ever since then I haven't had a day off school and I don't even get nervous any more if we have any tests. Mum keeps in contact with this lady and I feel better because in a way she is watching over me and keeping me healthy even though I've never met her. Mum has even had the dog treated like this as well.'

Gary Prosser

Reflexology

Origins

Various forms of foot massage were used in India, China and Egypt some 5,000 years ago, and were also popular amongst native American Indians and African tribespeople. Then, in 1913, Dr William Fitzgerald, an American ear, nose and throat surgeon at Boston General Hospital described 'zone therapy', precursor of modern reflexology. He apparently noticed that the application of pressure on focal points on the hands or feet could produce partial anaesthesia of areas in the ear, nose and throat. He went on to carry out minor surgical procedures using this method in place of more powerful conventional anaesthetics. He hypothesized that the body could be divided into 10 vertical zones, and that pressure on any one area within a certain zone was capable of having an influence on every other region in the same zone. Various followers took up this idea, including Doreen Bayley, who introduced reflexology to Britain in the 1960s, and set up the Bayley's School of Reflexology in 1968.

What is reflexology?

Reflexology is a therapy that involves the application of pressure to focal points on the feet or hands to encourage the body to heal from within. The term 'reflexology' stems from the idea that the therapy is derived from some kind of reflex action. Conventional physicians understand the term 'reflex' to have a specific meaning regarding one physiological aspect of the nervous system. In the knee-jerk reflex, for example, sharp stimulation of the quadriceps tendon with a reflex hammer just below the knee-cap sends sensory signals along afferent nerve fibres to the spinal cord, and back again along efferent, or motor pathways, resulting in contraction of the quadriceps muscle and a knee jerk. Reflexologists believe that applying pressure to a certain point on the sole of the foot, for example, will stimulate energy and healing in the body by having a distant effect on all other regions in the particular zone associated with that point. They go further, claiming that stimulation of reflexology points can also improve mental and physical health by having a general effect on the functioning of the autonomic nervous system. In this way, reflexologists claim to be able to promote harmonious digestion, calm anxiety and regularize breathing for example. Reflexology treatment mainly involves the practitioner applying his or her thumb or finger to points on the sole of the foot where pressure is applied to alter these physiological pathways in other parts of the body.

How does it work?

The basic tenet of reflexology is that all the body's organs and functions are represented in the soles of the feet. By applying pressure to specific areas on the feet, alteration to the functions of all the major organs of the body elsewhere can be brought about. The feet are seen as a kind of holographic mirror of the body, the concept being that small areas on the sole of each foot represent tiny microcosms of the larger organs situated elsewhere in the body. Consequently, if someone were to lie flat on their back with their toes pointing upwards, the view of the soles of their feet from the foot of the bed would be, a representative view of their entire body. The toes at the top would correspond to areas in the head and neck, the balls of the feet would be linked to the chest, lungs and shoulders, the arch of the foot would reflect the diaphragm, waist and pelvic area, and the heels would be mirrors of the sciatic nerve. Further territorial divisions on the sole of each foot are thought to correspond to more precise organ representation in the body, and are drawn up on special reflexology foot charts which are used by reflexologists.

Whether or not energy can really be rebalanced or stimulated from distant parts of the body by applying pressure to the foot, there is no doubt that many people benefit from the soothing and calming effect of foot massage. However, devotees of the practice claim that reflexology is not just ordinary foot massage. They even cite studies which have compared groups of patients receiving ordinary foot massage to other groups receiving reflexology. Their results suggest that specific reflexology is far more beneficial in achieving clinical results. Reflexologists would also claim that the additional relaxation effect is a bonus, and this is why pregnant women, people with chronic diseases like arthritis, people suffering with anxiety-related disorders, and even the terminally ill, derive such huge benefit from receiving it, and why more conventionally trained doctors and NHS hospitals are opening their doors as well as their minds to its clinical benefits.

According to the theory of zone therapy and the idea that the feet are windows of the body, someone complaining of a cold or sinusitis would have reflexology to the tops of their toes because this area corresponds to the head and sinus area on the reflexology foot chart. Some specialists claim that they can even diagnose and treat kidney or bladder problems by palpating the corresponding areas on the soles of the feet. Like other masseurs, reflexologists can sometimes detect tiny areas which feel like sand-grains, which they attribute to crystalline deposits of calcium located at any one of the 70,000 nerve endings known to exist in the soles of the feet. According to the feel, they can diagnose weak or overactive areas in the body, and claim that they can bring about healing by using their thumbs and fingers to change the flow of energy.

Is reflexology effective?

Ask the vast majority of people who have experienced reflexology, and they will tell you it works. Patients often say that the only time they did not think about their illness while they were in hospital was when they were having reflexology, and people being treated on an out-patient basis find it marvellous for alleviating stress-related conditions and anxiety. Patients are also very enthusiastic about its profoundly calming and soothing effects.

Despite the fact that some reflexologists are not keen to treat pregnant women, some studies have shown that reflexology can reduce the need for pain relief in labour, and that the second and most painful stage of labour itself could be shortened. A scientific study reported in the *Journal of Obstetrics and Gynaecology* also showed that the symptoms of premenstrual syndrome could also be significantly reduced by a hand, foot or ear reflexology session.

There is no known irrefutable scientific evidence that crystalline deposits, energy channels or 10 separate zones running vertically through the body actually exist, but there is evidence to show that stimulation of the nerve endings under the skin in one area of the body can produce pain and other sensations in deeper and distant regions. A child, with abdominal pain caused by appendicitis, for example, can have their pain eased by their mother stroking their tummy with a gentle warm hand. There is evidence, too, that biting hard on a dental wedge can help in tolerating severe pain. One explanation of this mechanism lies in the 'sensory gate' theory, which works on the principle that messages relaying pain along nerve fibres to one part of the spinal cord can be partially blocked by soothing and relaxing messages arriving along a different pathway from a different source, yet in the same zone and same site in the spinal cord.

What form might the treatment take?

A reflexology session usually lasts for about an hour, and is conducted in a welcoming and comfortable room, probably with some soothing music playing to create the right atmosphere. The patient is asked about their present symptoms and also about their previous medical and family history. They may also be asked if they are under any current treatment from their doctor or have any specific worries. Reflexology is normally practised with the patient lying back in a comfortable chair or on a couch. The bare feet are often wiped with tissue or cotton-wool soaked in witch-hazel but talcum powder or scented cream are alternatives. The practitioner usually starts with some relaxation techniques but will later dwell on specific problem areas and give them particular attention. The pressure applied is usually gentle, but deep thumb or finger pressure can certainly root out sensitive areas which the therapist may interpret as a sign of blocked energy in distant parts of the body. After treatment, the patient can feel a range of sensations. They may feel sleepy or drastically re-energized but should they feel light-headed or have any flu-like symptoms within two or three days, they can be reassured that these are not uncommon and may merely represent a signal that unbalanced energy is being adjusted and that problems are being overcome.

What problems are helped by reflexology?

Reflexology is really designed to boost energy levels and enhance emotional and spiritual well-being. The Association of Reflexologists specifically frowns on therapists diagnosing conditions, prescribing treatment or making improbable claims that they can remedy specific physical disorders. What reflexology certainly is effective at dealing with are stress-related conditions such as tension headaches, migraine, high blood pressure, irritable bowel syndrome, Raynaud's phenomenon, asthma and skin disorders such as psoriasis and eczema. It is also useful in treating back pain, general fatigue, menstrual irregularities, and even common disorders in childhood such as glue ear and night terrors. It is also useful in pregnancy where different kinds of relaxation technique, including breathing exercises, are known to be of benefit, and in terminal illness where the diagnosis itself is terrifying, and the side effects of powerful modern medicine, such as constipation and nausea can be so unpleasant. Reflexology is particularly useful for those patients who feel isolated, marginalized and depressed. An hour's relaxing massage at anyone's hands must, for them, be like manna from heaven – warm, close, soothing and deeply relaxing.

Is it safe?

Cautious reflexologists may be reluctant to treat patients suffering from diabetes or epilepsy, pregnant women or anyone receiving potent medication for particularly serious conditions. However, with everyone's consent, including that of the patient's doctor, the reflexologist can treat patients of all ages and in any state of health. Even children can enjoy short reflexology treatments although the feet of babies and toddlers require only the gentlest pressure with the thumb.

How can I find a reflexologist?

The British Reflexology Association (BRA) was established in 1985 and stemmed from the Bayley's School which was originally set up in 1968. Members use the letters MBRA (Member of the BRA) after their names. In addition, the Association of Reflexologists (AR) runs nearly 70 courses throughout the UK, to train its own professional reflexologists, who use the initials MAR (Member of the AR) after their name when they have qualified. Members of both organizations abide by a code of practice and ethics, and all registered members must carry professional indemnity. Local accredited therapists can be found through application to either establishment.

How much will it cost?

You can expect to pay about £25 for a session of reflexology, depending on where you live, but increasingly you may be offered reflexology as a luxury option as an in-patient of either an NHS or a private hospital.

The sceptic's view

The sceptic knows very well how wonderful an enthusiastic foot massage can be, but is it any more effective than an enthusiastic hair-do or any more therapeutic than a good manicure, or an afternoon of recreational shopping at Harrods? These, too, are good for one's emotional well-being, if not one's pocket, and may well re-vitalize and unblock energy channels. The disbeliever might also wonder why the pressure of a therapists thumb or finger might be any more effective than the pressure on the soles of the feet that results from normal walking. Why doesn't walking barefoot on an uneven surface cause all sorts of havoc among internal organs elsewhere in the body if the theory of reflexology holds water? Furthermore, how many reflexologists would come up with the same diagnosis for the same patient if they were not able to liaise and discuss the case together. At least if 10 conventionally trained doctors examined the same patient with the same enlarged liver, 90 per cent of them might detect the physical signs and come to a correct clinical conclusion. The sceptic doubts whether 10 unacquainted reflexologists could do the same.

The sceptic would also view the reflexologist's tenet that areas of tenderness represent energy blockages as being ridiculously convenient. Evoking further tenderness through massage is much more likely to leave an impression on the patient than rubbing non-sensitive areas to no effect whatsoever. A true doubting Thomas might quote with relish from one reflexology therapist's leaflet: 'After a treatment you may well feel exhausted or absolutely filled with energy, it depends entirely on you.' This is tantamount to saying: 'My therapy can have any effect whatsoever and is entirely unpredictable. But whatever it does, it must be good and I claim the credit for it as an effective reflexologist.' The same leaflet also states 'You may feel that you get worse before you get better. This occurs if your body is overcoming an infection or struggling against an underlying ailment.' Again, the raw translation of this runs: 'If my treatment makes you worse, it still isn't my fault. When you feel better in the future, you can thank me for what I've done.' However, the reflexology dissenter would probably pause and think about all those sweaty, smelly feet with which these willing complementary therapists are happy to spend an hour. Only then might the medically trained dissenter acknowledge that reflexology certainly has a place!

The therapist's view

'Before deciding to become a reflexologist, I experienced many other complementary therapies but was definitely "drawn" to the feet. It was a complete change in career from administration in art and book publishing and my love of feet has given me enormous satisfaction. So many clients have become more contented and more in control of their own lives.

'In my practice I have come across many conditions but most, if not all, are stress-related. Reflexology does not aim for a "cure", but I have found that it relieves, for example back pain, stiff necks, irritable bowel syndrome, headaches and poor skin conditions. I have even seen a definite improvement in a case of Bell's palsy. I would particularly mention a case of endometriosis. The client was a ski instructor due to be married six months after her first visit and was threatened with an operation to help her condition. With weekly sessions of reflexology and a careful diet, the bloating in her stomach ceased, her periods returned to normal, and she no longer experienced the fearful pain – no operation was needed.

'I cannot help being enthusiastic about reflexology. I work with a particularly gentle touch. The clients' calm faces, their comments – "walking on air", "never felt so relaxed", "I feel so revitalized" – daily bringing a feeling of thankfulness that I found my way into such a wonderful therapy.'

Elizabeth Fraser

The patient's view

'I have been receiving reflexology treatments for the last three years. It works particularly well for me. When I remember back to my first consultation – the uncomfortable areas of my feet, the heat and perspiration which occurred – I realize that my body is now more balanced. My treatments are relaxing and through the various zones of my feet my therapist and I can detect problem areas if they arise. There are so many aspects which contribute to good health. I see reflexology as a beneficial treatment to enhance inner health.'

J. Hallum

Relaxation and Visualization

Origins

Relaxation is a skill that everyone should master. It's a vital element in leading a healthy lifestyle, and its benefits are many and varied. Its importance has been recognized for centuries as part of the Eastern philosophies, and nowadays more and more people in the West are beginning to practise relaxation techniques. This includes the conventional medical profession, who are becoming increasingly aware of the advantages relaxation has for their patients.

In recent years a new area of medical research called psycho-neuro immunology has done much to reinforce the concept that conscious control within the brain can have a direct and powerful effect on the body, and vice versa. Some scientists even believe that thought-control can fight cancer cells and overcome infection through its enhancing effect on the immune system. Whilst this is an extreme view, many doctors believe that positive thinking and avoiding stress go a long way towards preventing ill-health.

What is relaxation and visualization?

The opposite of the stress response is the relaxation response, which in biological terms is every bit as important. It involves the part of the nervous system which slows our heart-beat, regulates our breathing, warms our skin and smoothly controls digestive processes. It brings about sleep and a sense of peace and tranquillity. It is a much more passive response than the stress response, however, and in a world where human beings are perpetually being put under strain and pressure, we have to work hard at promoting relaxation by switching off the stress response and allowing the body to relax and return to its natural rhythm. The techniques are useful in easing muscular tension, which brings about headaches and migraine; it helps reduce blood pressure and blood cholesterol levels; it is of benefit in circulatory disorders where blood-flow to the skin is restricted, as in Raynaud's phenomenon.

Relaxation and visualization are two distinct entities but are often merged into a single therapy. Relaxation is largely a stress-busting technique where apprehension, panic and tension can be alleviated. Visualization involves using one's imagination to conjure up happy and positive images which can be used to enhance relaxation and overcome psychological and emotional difficulties. People suffering from panic attacks, for example, can learn to visualize a tranquil scene from their past, such as a warm sandy beach on a sunny day. The more they concentrate on this scene, the more they are able to relax and allay the fear connected with their immediate surroundings or situation. Regular practice of this technique enables them to overcome their fears and apprehensions very effectively. People can learn to visualize the achievement of success, too. Athletes and other sports persons, actors and students about to take exams can all achieve more by visualizing themselves breaking the tape at the end of the race, receiving a standing ovation in the theatre or being awarded their final degree.

How does it work?

Part of the body's nervous system is under voluntary control. The rest, the 'involuntary' or 'autonomic' nervous system, works at a subconscious level, and involves the interplay between the 'sympathetic' branch, which gears us up for action, and the 'parasympathetic' branch, which brings about relaxation. We need the sympathetic system for the fight or flight response which kicks in when we are threatened or challenged and put in the situation of being hyper-alert, but we also need the parasympathetic system, which controls normal digestive processes, secretions from glands, and restores the heart-beat and respiratory rate to normal resting levels. Through relaxation and visualization, the parasympathetic nervous system can become more dominant, switching off the stress response which can otherwise do so much harm to the body if left overcharged all the time. By achieving this, the muscles relax, the mind is free from worries and anxieties, digestion improves, breathing becomes more even and efficient, the heart rate slows, the skin feels warmer, and aggression and irritability fade away.

Visualization is thought to work by stimulating the right side of the brain in particular. There are two hemispheres in the brain: the left side is concerned mainly with logic, analysis, word ability and reason, while the right side is largely the seat of creativity, fantasy, lateral thought, imagination and emotions. Most of the time, when we are working and going about our daily living, we use the left side, and the right side is fairly dormant. When we do use the right side, however, energies which are created within it can quite dramatically change the physical responses in the body, so that, for example, memories of any kind which we call up can profoundly alter the way we react and function. Visualization employs the creation of positive images which overcome the stress-inducing effects of left-brain function, and enable relaxation to occur. In this way, the insertion of positive, imaginary ideas can encourage the patient to achieve attainable goals, always provided, of course, that those goals remain realistic.

Are relaxation and visualization techniques effective?

These techniques can be extremely effective for everyone, but especially for those who are ambitious, driven, conscientious high achievers. These people tend to find it difficult to relax and switch off from work, and have several of the classical type-A personality characteristics which pre-programme them to a vulnerability to heart attacks, migraines, digestive disorders and aggression. Another group which responds very well to these techniques are the born worriers of this world, who are naturally nervous and tense, underconfident and prone to anxiety, insomnia and panic. Studies carried out in recent years have shown the technique to be of benefit to patients with tension headaches and inflammatory bowel disease, and even to patients with Raynaud's phenomenon. This is a condition where hypersensitivity of the blood vessels in the fingers and toes to cold weather produces stiff, painful, numb, white fingers. By combining visualization and biofeedback techniques, patients with this condition can learn to overcome the overactivity of the sympathetic nervous system, which triggers the Raynaud's phenomenon, and benefit considerably. With biofeedback, a patient under stress learns to recognize how their thought processes, pulse, respiration, blood pressure and temperature all respond to tension. By linking one with the other they can apply relaxation techniques to actively control these functions whenever it is appropriate

What form might the treatment take?

Therapy can take place in groups or on an individual basis. Sessions will last a minimum of 45 minutes as time is required to fully relax, but before therapy starts, a medical history will be taken so that the therapist can tailor the techniques to the individual's need. It is possible that skin temperature, pulse rate and blood pressure may be examined, but this of course depends on the level of qualification of the practitioner. Patients will be asked to make themselves comfortable, either sitting or lying on a couch or on the floor, and then the therapist will begin the individual relaxation exercises. They come in a variety of forms, and the therapist takes the patient through the ones with which he or she is most familiar.

The exercises can, of course, be done at home, and even a complete beginner who has not seen a therapist can enjoy them. Before you begin, you should prepare for relaxation in the following way:

How to prepare for relaxation

1. Find a quiet place where you will not be disturbed by anybody or the telephone. Make sure this place is warm as well as quiet.
2. Sit in a comfortable chair with both feet flat on the floor relaxing your shoulders and sinking back into the chair which supports you.
3. Slip off your shoes and rest your arms on your lap.
4. Consciously slow your rate of breathing, taking deep, regular breaths.
5. Breathe out for twice as long as you breathe in, controlling the rhythm by silently counting to yourself.
6. Close your eyes and, as you continue to breathe rhythmically, clear your mind of all thoughts and worries.
7. Carry on with the deep breathing, concentrating now on where the muscular tensions are in your body.
8. Stop the deep breathing at any time if you begin to feel dizzy.
9. Breathe in through your nose and out through your mouth, expanding your abdomen as you inhale and raising your rib cage to allow more air to flow in, until your lungs feel completely filled. Hold your breath for five or six seconds before breathing out again slowly, allowing your rib cage and stomach to relax, emptying your lungs totally.
10. Carry on with the breathing exercise for five minutes or so.
11. You are now ready to start a muscular relaxation technique but should you wish to concentrate on anything which you know will relax you further then contemplate a while longer. Think about fond memories, happy events and wonderful holidays. Concentrate on events that have made you satisfied and fulfilled in the past. This combination of thinking relaxing thoughts and deep slow breathing means that the next step will be even more effective.

Having established a regular breathing pattern, you are now ready to start the next procedure, namely progressive muscular relaxation:

Progressive muscular relaxation

Using the following steps as a guide, start tensing the different parts of the body, one after the other, as you breathe in. Hold your breath for five seconds while you keep the muscles tense, then relax and breathe out again slowly over about ten seconds.

1 Curl your toes right up and press down with your feet, then relax.
2 Press your heels down, pulling your toes up. Relax.
3 Tense your calf muscles. Relax.
4 Straighten your legs and tense your thigh muscles. Relax.
5 Tighten your buttocks. Relax.
6 Tighten up your stomach muscles. Relax.
7 Bend your elbows up and flex your biceps. Relax.
8 Hunch your shoulders and tense your neck muscles. Relax.
9 Clench your teeth, frown and screw up your eyes as tight as you can. Relax.
10 Tense all your muscles at the same time and, after ten seconds, relax.
11 Close your eyes. Concentrate your mind on an imaginary diamond glinting on a black velvet background for 30 seconds as you continue to breathe slowly and deeply.
12 Focus on another peaceful object of your choice for 30 seconds.
13 Open your eyes.

This technique is designed to help you recognize muscular tension in your body so that you can learn to relax it at will. The more the technique is practised, the easier this will become and you can do it in the car, in the office, on the bus, practically anywhere.

Visualization not only helps people overcome tension, fear and stress, it can also enhance concentration and alertness, giving memory and creativity a boost at the same time. Once the patient is fully relaxed, the therapist is often able to guide the visualization exercises away from anxiety-provoking thoughts in the patient towards more positive calming images which, in turn, will enable the unpleasant symptoms of tension and anxiety to be overcome. The patient needs to practise visualization for at least 15 minutes every day so that a calming reflex can be established which can be called upon whenever needed.

What problems are helped by relaxation and visualization?

Since these techniques abolish muscular tension, both headaches and migraines can be alleviated. They also reduce blood pressure and even blood cholesterol levels, and are of benefit in circulatory disorders where blood flow to the skin is restricted, for example in Raynaud's phenomenon. These techniques are also useful for treating arthritis, irritable bowel syndrome, anxiety states, panic attacks, sleeping disorders and a host of other physical conditions. Mental well-being is improved as well, concentration is boosted and many people find that their memory and creativity are enhanced. Above all, relaxation means that people can become less dependent on artificial sedatives such as tranquillizers, antidepressants and hypnotic drugs. It provides welcome relief from the turmoil and chaos going on around us, and an opportunity for the human body and spirit to recharge their exhausted batteries.

Is it safe?

By and large, relaxation and visualization techniques are safe for everybody including pregnant women, the elderly and small children. However, they should be used with caution by people whose blood pressure is already low, such as people who have suffered a stroke or are on certain medications. People with inflammatory arthritis will not be comfortable lying still on a hard surface for any length of time. Whilst the techniques can be used for the mentally ill, they should only be carried out under the supervision of a therapist trained in mental health, and since they sometimes induce a feeling of fatigue, patients who are already tired from conditions such as ME (myalgic encephalomyelitis) or terminal disease should be wary. The techniques focus on usually subconscious functions, such as the pulse and breathing, and some patients have reported 'heart-consciousness' after treatment, when the patient is unable to stop being aware of every heart-beat or of how deep or shallow, rapid or fast their breathing has become. Generally speaking, however, relaxation and visualization techniques are beneficial to all patients and if the population at large practised them, the world would undoubtedly be a calmer more peaceful and sympathetic place to live in.

How can I find a relaxation therapist?

Since there are no statutory qualifications for people using these techniques, it may be difficult to know where to find help. Many practitioners use the techniques along with other complementary therapies and many will be on the British Register of Complementary Practitioners. However, some hospital-based occupational therapists use these techniques, as do many nurses and doctors, as part of their therapeutic repertoire. Many clinical psychologists, hypnotists and psychotherapists also use the methods in addition to their mainstream work. Your doctor may be able to recommend somebody locally, or you might know someone who has benefited. Beware of therapists advertising in the Yellow Pages who are not known to you at all.

What will it cost?

In some areas patients can obtain treatment under the NHS. Otherwise, private therapy will usually cost anything between £20 and £60 per session, depending on the qualifications and experience of the therapist and the area in which you live.

The sceptic's view

The sceptic doubts whether a born worrier could ever be made less anxious by practising these techniques, and suspects that spending hours trying to master visualization or deep muscular relaxation, only to find that they don't help, could do more harm than good to an already panic-prone patient. The level of control any of us has over our autonomic nervous system is strictly limited, and far more significant effects can be achieved using safe, modern pharmaceutical preparations: the heart rate can be significantly slowed by beta-blockers; the skin circulation can be enhanced for people with Raynaud's phenomenon using vasodilators; and the spasm within the intestinal wall in patients with irritable bowel syndrome can be improved using antispasmodics. Lying around thinking pleasant thoughts is all very well, but how many stressed-out individuals have really got time for it?

The therapist's view

'I never cease to be amazed by how much can be achieved through this therapy. It seems to me that people have simply lost the art of being aware of the effects of stress in their lives, and have forgotten how to recognize the physical and emotional consequences of it. I have treated people who cannot sleep, who have panic attacks, who have chronic asthma, who take handfuls of tablets for blood pressure, and whose palpitations alarm them enormously. After just one session, either in a group or on a one-to-one basis, they often feel happier about themselves and begin to develop an understanding of what their bodies are telling them. After several sessions they are enthusiastic about practising relaxation and visualization regularly, and without any encouragement are singing its praises to friends and relatives, often inviting them to join the group. The therapy is rewarding because it means people are able to reduce the medication they take (with the permission of their family doctors, I hasten to add), and can learn to control the unpleasant symptoms of an overactive intestine, an over-stimulated nervous system, and a cardiovascular system which is over-stressed. I see people around town who have been clients of mine in the past, and almost all of them are still using the technique they learned from me in one form or another.'

D. Allum

The patient's view

'My problem is Raynaud's phenomenon which gives me very cold extremities, even when the weather is only relatively cool. It is a sensitivity of the blood vessels in my fingers and toes, which means that they go numb and blue and are very painful when they start to thaw out again. I didn't like the idea of taking tablets every day, as my doctor suggested, so I learned how to use visualization as a method of helping my problem. I learned a technique called "biofeedback", which enabled me to train my body to "think itself warm" simply by visualizing myself in a hot bath or lying in the hot sand of the Sahara desert. People think it's crazy, but even on cold days now, if I think myself really warm, my fingers and toes do not suffer so much.'

Claudine Bowman

Shiatsu

Origins

Shiatsu originated in Japan and, very much like traditional Chinese medicine was devised as a holistic therapy for improving physical, emotional and spiritual health. Shiatsu is the modern version of Amma, an ancient massage therapy used to treat common medical complaints through manipulation of the body by rubbing and pressing. Shiatsu became firmly established in Japan in the seventeenth century, but in the last 100 years has incorporated some of the techniques of chiropractic and osteopathy, which have helped to make it one of the commonest and most widely practised forms of treatment in Japan today. It was brought to Britain in the late 1970s and in 1981 the Shiatsu Society was founded.

What is shiatsu?

Literally translated, shiatsu means 'finger pressure'. In addition to the fingers, however, the therapist uses thumbs, elbows, arms, knees and feet to move and position the patient's body and to apply pressure to certain points known as 'tsubos' scattered about the body's main energy channels. In this respect it is like acupuncture without needles but the increased emphasis on massage and therapeutic touch enables shiatsu to bring the therapist and the patient closer together.

How does it work?

Shiatsu is based on the principle that ill-health is brought about by abnormalities in the flow of energy within the body. It shares the same methods of diagnosis and the belief in 12 energy channels or meridians with traditional Chinese medicine (see pages 103–5). The patient's energy may be diminished ('kyo') or enhanced and overactive ('jitsu'). By applying pressure at the acupoints, the shiatsu therapist aims to correct any abnormal interruptions to this energy flow, or 'ki'.

Is shiatsu effective?

There is no doubt that, by and large, the recipient of shiatsu finds it surprisingly effective, particularly for stress-related disorders and for back and neck problems. However, at present very little objective scientific evidence exists that quantifies any benefits. One Chinese study found it to be dramatically effective in treating chronic low back pain in car workers who were not only rendered pain free, but who reported improved sleep as an additional bonus. Another double blind trial, published in the *Journal of the Royal Society of Medicine*, showed that shiatsu improved morning sickness in women attending the Royal Maternity Hospital in Belfast. Another study, conducted by the Shiatsu Society itself in 1992, stated that shiatsu is even useful in controlling thalamic pain seen in a rare condition where physiological damage occurs in a deep-seated part of the brain called the thalamus, which itself is responsible for the transmission of pain sensations along nerve pathways. Notoriously difficult to treat by conventional methods, several sufferers of this condition found shiatsu useful, not only in relieving pain, but also in helping them to relax, and the majority continued to use it on a regular basis thereafter.

What form might the treatment take?

A first consultation with a shiatsu therapist can be anything from 30 minutes to an hour and a half long. In order to attempt to establish a diagnosis, the therapist will ask the patient about their current health and their medical history. He or she will be particularly interested in the patient's lifestyle and relationships, the kind of work they do, what they eat and how much exercise they take. The therapist will then observe and palpate parts of the patient's body to gain further clues as to the underlying problem. It is not necessary to undress for the session, but because of the nature of the manipulation, unrestrictive clothing is recommended.

The patient is likely to be asked to lie down on a futon while the therapist gently palpates the abdomen or 'hara', which is regarded as the 'ocean of ki'. This is perhaps the most important part of the overall examination. The treatment itself consists of the therapist massaging, stretching, rubbing and squeezing parts of the body at both deep and superficial levels in an attempt to correct any disturbances of energy flow. Pressure will be applied to the 'tsubos' using the therapist's own hands, elbows or knees. Although this is designed to relax, it may also bring about a slight discomfort or pleasurable pain. Patients should be warned that although most people feel refreshed after their therapy, some can experience headaches or flu-like symptoms for up to 24 hours afterwards. These are interpreted as encouraging signs that toxins or energy blockages have been released. For particular health complaints or emotional problems, one session or so a month is often recommended, but for chronic conditions patients may eventually be taught a DIY technique known as 'do-in'. Essentially, this is a form of shiatsu based on self-stimulation.

What problems are helped by shiatsu?

Shiatsu specialists use the technique to improve general well-being, for stress relief and for allaying anxiety. It also seems to be particularly useful for back and neck pain and the associated headaches and insomnia they may bring about. It is also used to treat disorders of the digestive system, and because of its usefulness in the musculo-skeletal area it is often used for relief of physical disabilities such as cerebral palsy and strokes. It is now used in some NHS cancer wards and drug rehabilitation centres, and a growing number of HIV-positive patients seem to derive benefit from it.

Is it safe?

Shiatsu involves the physical manipulation of the patient, so it should not be used to treat patients with osteoporosis or brittle bone disease or women in the early stages of pregnancy. Generally speaking, however, the technique is safe and the Shiatsu Society maintains that no complaints about this form of therapy have been received.

How can I find a shiatsu practitioner?

Shiatsu has only recently been introduced in the UK, and there are still only a handful of practitioners, the vast majority of whom belong to the Shiatsu Society. Make sure that any shiatsu practitioner you see is a Registered Member of the Shiatsu Society (RMSS) and is governed by its code of practice and ethics. If you fail to do this, you are not taking adequate precautions against becoming the victim of improper or inappropriate treatment or conduct, and you will be less able to satisfy yourself with any legal comeback.

How much will it cost?

Each session will cost in the region of £25 but the price will vary from therapist to therapist and area to area.

The sceptic's view

The sceptic would point out the lack of medical qualifications of many shiatsu practitioners and scoff at their form of diagnosis, which they admit relies to a large extent on intuition. The cynic would also make short shrift of those mysterious energy channels and 'tsubos', and would stress that the mere fact that the patient does not even have to get undressed for the examination shows that it is neither a thorough nor a reliable medical practice.

The therapist's view

'Shiatsu enjoys a long and distinguished history in Japan where it was first practised as a preventative therapy. Its roots can be traced back to a form of body work called Amma, first discussed in *The Yellow Emperor's Classic* 2,000 years ago. Shiatsu has moved on from Amma whilst keeping faithful to the tenets of oriental medicine.

'Shiatsu is a deeply relaxing therapy that provides stimulation by applying natural pressure to the meridians (channels of energy that run along the body) and applies gentle stretches. It consists of a whole body treatment as it is believed that a disorder in one area can have effects elsewhere in the body.

'Shiatsu's popularity rests upon its effectiveness in treating a wide spectrum of disorders whilst being very pleasurable to receive. Its ability to rebalance and adjust the energy of the recipient, thereby relieving stress and tension, make it a very effective therapy for many modern-day problems, including disorders that affect the musculor-skeletal system; lymphatic and blood circulation; internal organ functions, and for calming the nervous system. Any symptoms or illnesses caused by malfunctions in any of these areas can be treated by shiatsu. As a preventative therapy it strengthens one's own innate curative resources to promote a healthier and more relaxed life.'

Nic Kyriacou
London College of Shiatsu

The patient's view

'The first thing you notice when you receive a shiatsu treatment is that all the nonsense stops. By that I mean that you lie, either on your front (prone) or back (supine), and all the ridiculous thoughts running through your head – about work, things to do, the bloke who cut you up on the road this morning – all evaporate one by one as the treatment gets underway.

'A wonderful feeling of calm takes the place of the "nonsense" as the practitioner diagnoses your current state of health. To do this they place their hand on your 'hara' (abdomen) where they can feel the fullness ("jitsu") or emptiness ("kyo") of each organ. According to their diagnosis, they balance the meridians which relate to every major organ in the body, and which run from the top of the head to the feet.

'This involves deep massage that quite often sends you to sleep – it cuts across all the body's defences, and by subtle manipulation, and sometimes co-ordinated breathing between practitioner and receiver, reduces all stiffness in joints and muscles.

'After a few sessions, you are able to realize yourself when you're tense in a particular area, and consequently work on relaxing that tension. You can also do shiatsu on yourself, and there are various reasonably priced books on self-shiatsu ("do-in") at large book stores.

'Whatever, to practise or receive shiatsu with any regularity, is to know and feel closer to the body that is trying its best to usher you through life.'

David Yates

Spiritual Healing

Origins

The origins of spiritual healing are found in black magic, voodooism and religion. In Christianity, Jesus was described as a healer, and certain geographical places are well known as centres of spiritual healing to which thousands of people still make regular pilgrimage. Lourdes is perhaps the best known example. In 1955, the National Federation of Spiritual Healers was established by Harry Edwards who believed he was an energy conduit for the healing powers of Joseph Lister and Louis Pasteur. Although Edwards's work was never accepted or endorsed by the orthodox medical fraternity, they did however go so far as to admit that the sporadic cases of healing in apparently hopeless medical cases did occasionally seem to take place without any rational basis in clinical science.

As membership of the federation grew, and more people came to be impressed with results of spiritual healing, the Department of Health decreed that interested NHS GPs could permit spiritual healers to practise within their premises on the proviso that clinical responsibility remained with the doctors. Today, there are over 7,000 spiritual healers registered in the UK with a few conventionally trained doctors even adopting the practice, and there are scores of healers working on NHS hospital wards with the full permission of the consultants in charge.

What is spiritual healing?

Spiritual healing involves the channelling of energy from a distant source through a healer's hands to any person who requires it. The source is considered by some to be divine, coming from God, but those without religious faith believe it is of cosmic or universal origin, and too powerful for any of us to understand. The treatment acts on both the body and the mind, and may be used to benefit patients with emotional, psychological or physical problems. Healing can be carried out through the laying on of hands, and may even be practised from a distance. There are a number of different types.

Spiritual healing

Spiritual healing generally implies the ancient tradition of laying on of hands. This does not require the patient or the therapist to have any religious faith, and can even be carried out at a distance, though generally at a prearranged time when the therapist conceptualizes the transmission of healing energy through themselves to the patient. The patient can physically be hundreds of miles away when this is carried out.

Faith healing

This type of healing is generally performed in a religious setting, often in prayer groups or within a church congregation.

Therapeutic touch

This is a form of spiritual healing for which the healer's hands do not actually touch the patient at all, but are held just over the surface of the body. Healers using this technique believe they can explore the patient's natural 'aura', or energy field, and can correct any detectable imbalance.

Reiki

This is a Japanese system of healing, which incorporates not only the laying on of hands, but light massage and distant healing procedures as well.

How does it work?

No one, not even the healers themselves, really knows the answer to this question. There is no universal agreement on the source of the healing energy, nor is it understood why some people seem to have a healing gift while others do not. The consensus of opinion is that every human being has their own flow of healing energy coursing around their body, which can become compromised in various circumstances. When healers employ their gift and apply their hands to a patient's body, they become a channel or conduit for the flow of healing energy which will restore harmony and equilibrium to the patient. Contrary to popular belief, however, the power of healing is not clearly black or white, capable only of curing or not curing; it can also help people cope with chronic illness or terminal disease, and just by making people feel better and more calm, can improve their quality of life.

Is spiritual healing effective?

Although the majority of doctors dismiss the idea of spiritual healing as nonsensical and superstitious mumbo-jumbo, some have been so impressed with its applications that they have joined the UK-based Doctor–Healer Network which is connected to the Confederation of Healing Organizations. Many scientific trials have been conducted on the effects of spiritual healing and some may be interpreted as showing positive results.

One of the more interesting on-going pieces of research involves a healer who has been seeing patients at a general practice surgery in the West Country, all of whom are suffering from chronic conditions which have not responded to conventional therapy. After the first six months of the project, some three-quarters of the patients reported an improvement in their symptoms. How much of this may be due to any placebo effect, however, is not clear but what does appear to be evident is that these patients benefited, and that this in turn freed up time for the GPs to see other patients.

Most GPs would agree that some kind of faith is important for many people, and it certainly helps them to come to terms with acute loss and bereavement, as well as to face death and dying more calmly. In fact, anything that improves the quality of a patient's life, whatever medical situation they are in, must surely be welcome. The 'missionary' healers who tour huge arenas internationally certainly need no further scientific proof of the benefits. Healers themselves, however, do not generally claim that they can 'cure' patients. Indeed, it would be foolish as well as dangerous if they did, as reputable healers would be the first to admit that healing does not work for everyone. More research is required to look into the long-term as well as the immediate effects of healing, but patients may very well feel encouraged, supported and improved after just one session with a charismatic healer. How long those effects last is unpredictable.

What form might the treatment take?

Healers may work in a religious setting, but more often than not, their therapy takes place at the patient's home, at a healing centre or even in NHS GP premises. Some healing is even delivered in the hospital environment. The treatment may be given on a one-to-one basis, or in a group, and the first session will normally take about an hour. The patient's current problems and treatment, and past history are probed, and a reputable healer will ask whether a doctor has already been consulted. He or she is generally much happier if they have.

For the therapy, the patient may be sitting or lying down, and they are asked to relax completely and close their eyes. As the healer's hands are applied to the skin, or just over the skin, patients may feel a hot sensation or experience pins and needles, which many find surprising. Even total disbelievers may be excited when this happens. Reactions after treatment vary from feeling energized and enlivened to feeling detached, light-headed and emancipated from their illness. Follow-up sessions will generally last 15–30 minutes and, depending on the symptoms experienced by the patient, several sessions may be recommended.

What problems are helped by spiritual healing?

Spiritual healing is promoted as a holistic therapy, and does not therefore confine itself to physical ailments. Disorders as diverse as backache, arthritis, heart disease, anxiety and depression, headaches, ME (myalgic encephalomyelitis), asthma, insomnia and many others may all be brought before the spiritual healer. Even chronic conditions and terminal illness come their way.

Is it safe?

Whilst spiritual healing is safe in itself, any concrete promises that the patient may be cured or even vastly improved can unfairly raise hopes in the patient whose disappointment could be enormous should the therapy fail. This could have far-reaching consequences, including suicide. No self-respecting healer should make promises or guarantees, nor claim to be able to cure any specific condition. Any current medication the patient is taking should be continued and the patient's doctor should always be consulted. Healers should also point out that because the effects are unpredictable and may release unresolved emotions and feelings, patients may sometimes feel worse before they notice any improvement. This is in keeping with many complementary therapies, which can have similar results when internal healing displaces inner disharmony and draws it towards the surface.

How can I find a spiritual healer?

The biggest umbrella organization is the Confederation of Healing Organizations (CHO), which consists of a number of different groups and boasts several thousand members. The biggest single group within it is the National Federation of Spiritual Healers, incorporating healers from Christian, Buddhist and non-religious backgrounds. Members of the CHO abide by a recognized code of ethics which prevents healers from claiming to perform miracles and cures, and encourages patients not to lose confidence in their orthodox medical treatment and to keep their doctors informed as to what they are doing. Members are insured for the work they carry out, and it is proposed that in the future some form of nationally recognized qualification will be required. There are, of course, healers who are not part of any organization, and indeed there are no academic qualifications in spiritual healing. Hysterical evangelistic healers are best avoided, and large sums of money should never change hands in return for treatment.

How much will it cost?

Some healers make no charge at all for their services as they do not seek to make a profit from their 'gift', which they themselves interpret as a gift from God. Others merely ask for a contribution to be made towards their expenses, but very few healers ask for more than £30–40 for the first session. Occasionally, healing may be obtained on the NHS if the GP fund-holder is willing to make the referral, or if the GP happens to be a healer themselves.

The sceptic's view

Here is shamanism and superstition at their worst. Fooling the gullible public into believing that another human being can magically improve their lot in life is shameful. There is no divine power that can influence disease through the laying on of hands, and this type of witchcraft does not stand up to scientific scrutiny. There are no miracle cures and the disappearance of widespread cancer or the spontaneous resolution of leukaemia has never been proved. There have been cases of mistaken diagnosis, of course, for which healers may have occasionally taken the credit, but there have also certainly been cases of people dying as a result of being told by their healer to discontinue their conventional treatment. Whether or not the patient feels any burning heat or pins and needles when the therapist applies his or her hands, or waves them about the patient's body, you might as well have your palms read by a blind alcoholic gypsy for all the good it might do. Many a devotee of spiritual healing has grudgingly crawled back to the conventional doctor asking to have their inflamed appendix removed or their broken limb splinted when for years they believed this could be mended through healing.

The therapist's view

'I believe that spiritual healing is the most empowering yet gentle form of therapy which mobilizes the patient's own healing energy to restore balance and order where there is disharmony and disease. It allows the person to take responsibility for his/her own well-being and to work hand in hand with the healer who acts merely as a conduit for the flow of energy. Healing is an active partnership between the therapist and the person asking for healing and, if able, the patient is encouraged to continue the healing after the formal session is over by the use of various techniques, including meditation and spiritual exercises. Healing always takes place, though the results may vary from a state of relaxation and peace, which allows the patient's own resources to be better utilized to a profound alteration in the physical, emotional and spiritual state, with a return to good health. It is the perfect therapy to use in conjunction with orthodox medical techniques if these are necessary, giving the patient the feeling of maintaining control.'

Dr Brenda Davies

The patient's view

'After several weeks of investigation, I was diagnosed as having cancer of the prostate, which unfortunately had already spread to the bones in my lower spine. I suffered from terrible back pain, which felt like somebody was twisting a cork-screw into the bone itself. I was on hormonal treatment and I had some radiotherapy but it was unbelievable how much pain I was in. Painkillers really knocked me out, and I didn't want to live the rest of my life spaced out. In desperation but with an open mind I went along to see a spiritual healer. When the healer touched my back I felt this amazing sensation of heat, which surprised me because I would never have believed it if I had not experienced it myself. For about 10 days afterwards I was relatively pain free, and although I still have some gnawing pain, it is nowhere near as bad as it used to be, and somehow I feel much better in myself about the future and the way I shall be able to cope with the difficulties ahead.'

David Hankin

T'ai chi

Origins

According to oriental folklore, t'ai chi was originated by the Taoist monk and martial arts expert, Chang San Feng, who lived during the Sung Dynasty of the twelfth century. Both a soldier and a spiritualist, Chang San Feng was apparently inspired to develop t'ai chi after watching a fascinating duel between a snake and a crane, during which the snake mesmerized, confused and finally overcame the more powerful and heavier bird by its artful and inscrutable speed and grace. According to popular legend, so impressed was Chang San Feng that he developed his own system of, non-combative martial art exercises that integrated the flexibility and versatility of the snake-like movements, along with relaxation, breathing exercises and meditation.

When China opened its doors to Westerners and allowed them to travel freely within its territories once again, the widespread practice of t'ai chi was evident for all to see. Every public place at dawn was full of people practising the familiar slow-motion movements and deliberate postures. From then on, t'ai chi was exported to the West where it has grown in popularity ever since the 1970s and where it continues to grow as a beautiful and soothing antidote to the stresses and strains of our mad, fraught and desensitized existence.

What is t'ai chi?

'T'ai chi chuan' literally means 'the supreme unity of the fist'. It is an ancient system of oriental medicine which combines a gentle martial art with meditation and a series of seamless exercises designed to enhance the health of the body and the mind. It also incorporates other Chinese therapies, such as acupuncture, herbal medicine and massage, and is influenced by Buddhist, Taoist and Confucian philosophies, all of which maintain that the two opposing energies of Yin and Yang operate throughout our universe (see pages 103–4).

How does it work?

Although there are many different styles of t'ai chi, they are all basically designed to assist the fluency of our vital energy and to help balance the ebb and flow of nature itself. Different varieties of exercise rhythms and postures may be adopted in different styles of t'ai chi. The Yang style, for example, is slow and strong, consisting of large open gestures, while the Chen style intersperses calm, slow movements with sudden, rapid, coiling, snake-like movements. Developed from basic self-defence postures, t'ai chi movements are given names which are aggressive sounding, such as 'punch with hidden fist' or 'kick with left heel', although t'ai chi is neither competitive nor combative. It can be practised alone or in a class, and its slow, fluid, sequential movements are designed to promote harmony and calm in the continuum of the mind, body and soul. It aims to restore equilibrium to the energy flow which courses through the meridian channels in the body, and because it incorporates relaxation, breathing and thought exercises, it has been dubbed by some 'meditation in motion'. T'ai chi is practised as a form of complete relaxation for both the nervous and the musculo-skeletal systems of the body. It is promoted as a practice that improves posture and enhances the immune system whilst stimulating the circulation and lymphatic channels of the body, and boosting suppleness and respiratory function at the same time.

Is t'ai chi effective?

T'ai chi is really a preventative health practice, and it is therefore difficult to find scientific evidence to prove that it works. As a form of therapy, however, which combines coordination, balance, abstract and creative thought, meditation and breathing exercises, it is a wonderful way to combat stress, and as such, can be of benefit to millions who have stress-related disorders. Its very widespread adoption in Britain bears testimony to its appeal and popularity, and the high regard that many people working in health care now have for it. Many a patient rehabilitating from long-standing disorders such as arthritis, or even heart attack, may be seen practising this fascinating therapy in any of Britain's public places at all hours of the day and night.

What form might the treatment take?

T'ai chi is usually taught in classes of 20 or so people. Classes generally last about an hour and a half, and loose, comfortable clothes, such as leotards or track suits, are worn. After 15 minutes of warm-up exercises, the class then goes on to 'learn a form'. The short form of t'ai chi involves movements that can be conducted in about 10 minutes, and the long form can take anything up to 40 minutes to an hour. It can take a year to learn a short form, and much longer to learn the long form, because each movement has to be perfected, and the sequence of the movements, which must flow gently into one another, has to be remembered. Because of this, it is generally a harder discipline to master than yoga.

What problems are helped by t'ai chi?

T'ai chi is particularly good at helping tension, anxiety and any stress-related disorders, such as skin complaints, stomach ulcers, headaches, high blood pressure and circulatory problems. It can be of enormous benefit to people with rheumatic complaints, and patients recovering from injuries or accidents, and its gentle nature makes it particularly suitable for the rehabilitation of people recovering from heart attacks or even from heart or lung surgery. Flexibility can be one of the benefits of t'ai chi, and for this reason, people with stiffness due to low back pain or osteoporosis can reap rewards from learning the art. In addition, people with physical difficulties such as multiple sclerosis, muscular dystrophy and neuritis, and even those confined to wheelchairs, may genuinely benefit from t'ai chi.

Is it safe?

Provided the teacher of t'ai chi is experienced and qualified, and knows about any relevant medical problem his pupil may have, t'ai chi is a gentle and safe exercise system for people of any age, irrespective of their level of health and fitness.

How can I find a t'ai chi teacher?

Anyone interested in learning t'ai chi should ask their local authority about evening classes, and fitness clubs about any courses they run.

How much will it cost?

Generally speaking, a t'ai chi class will cost in the region of £5–10, but because several sessions are required as a basic minimum to make any satisfactory improvement, special rates are often offered for 10–20 sessions at a time.

The sceptic's view

The Western cynic might argue that if God had wanted us to act like a snake, he would have given us a forked tongue, a scaly skin and a rattle in our tail. He or she might well regard many of the postures and movements of t'ai chi as unnatural, and query the suitability of these slow laborious animal-mimicking exercises that are far too time-consuming and ridiculous for our sophisticated and civilized modern world.

Conventional doctors are definitely sold on the idea of rehabilitation for patients but they would almost certainly prefer them to pedal for hours on an exercise bike or a rowing machine, rather that standing on one leg with both arms in the air looking like a praying mantis about to eat its mate.

The therapist's view

'I've been practising t'ai chi for an hour a day, come rain or shine, for over 20 years now, and am just beginning to scratch beneath the surface of this ancient arcane art. No matter how fragile or worse for wear I feel from the night before, a round or two of the t'ai chi form, or warrior dance, rejuvenates and refreshes me.

'Through the gentle stretching motions I have overcome back and shoulder pains, colds and flus, and generally boosted my immune system. The energy or chi generated affords me enormous stamina in my everyday life, gives me confidence and has also enabled me to heal others. The martial or boxing aspect of the art increases my mental concentration and focus and lends grace and fluidity to my movements throughout my working day. As well as these advantages of suppleness and flexibility, the practice has enabled me to find peace of mind and equipoise amidst the hectic to-ing and fro-ing of my busy life as a professional healer, author, journalist, composer and martial arts teacher (no kidding!).

'T'ai chi is easy and effortless to learn if you're willing to give it the time, and is suitable for young and old alike. In fact it gets better as you get older. For myself, I believe t'ai chi has saved my life in more ways than one. It is exhilarating to perform, similar, I'd imagine, to flying free like a bird, and if it sounds like I'm given to hyperbole, it's simply because I think t'ai chi is one of the cleverest inventions yet developed by humankind. I recommend it highly.'

Stephen Russell
(The barefoot doctor)

The patient's view

'After spending the last 20 years of my life as a businessman travelling backwards and forwards from the Far East and London, I suffered a heart attack at the age of 58. Physically, I made a good recovery, but the thing I found hardest to overcome was the lack of confidence about what I could and couldn't do in the future. I used to worry about walking the dog, I avoided taking the grandchildren out lest I collapsed whilst looking after them, and all in all I became something of a cardiac cripple. Then a chance meeting with an ex-business associate in China introduced me to t'ai chi. I checked with my family doctor and was somewhat surprised when he enthusiastically encouraged me to give it a whirl. I went along to the classes, and within a few months was totally hooked. It made me feel both peaceful and relaxed, and for the first time in ages I began to experience a new vigour and energy which I thought I had permanently lost. My self-confidence returned, and whether it is a coincidence or not, I have been able in recent weeks to reduce fairly significantly the amount of medication I take for my heart rate and blood pressure.'

Christopher Saunders

Yoga

Origins

Indian philosophers and yogis used meditation as part of their spiritual practises. It probably started some 5,000 years ago, several hundred years before the first known statues illustrating yogic postures were ever made. Yoga was probably first brought to Britain in the Victorian era, and it has become increasingly popular since the 1960s.

What is yoga?

Contrary to popular belief, yoga is not merely a relaxation system which contortionists can enjoy. In fact, it is a gentle discipline from which even the disabled, the arthritic, the elderly and the terminally ill can draw benefit. It is an exercise system which enhances the psyche as well as the soma; the word yoga is actually derived from the Sanskrit for 'union', and it is a way of promoting union between the mind and the body. Not only do the postures adopted in yoga aim to increase suppleness and strength, but the philosophy and relaxation is designed to alleviate stress and counter negative emotions, while at the same time promoting a healthy lifestyle. The inner calm and concentration which accompanies yoga enhances spiritual well-being whilst focusing the body on those functions which normally work beyond our conscious control, such as breathing and digestion, so that continual practice brings about an overall balance and harmony. When used regularly, yoga can therefore relieve complaints such as tension, anxiety, back pain, depression and arthritis. There are three main types of yoga: breathing, called Pranayama; the adoption of postures, called Asanas; meditation, known as Dhyana. Constant practice of these three elements is designed to allow the practitioner to reach total self-enlightenment and mastery of the body.

How does it work?

The union of mind and body is brought about by correct breathing, physical exercises and meditation. Tension, unhappiness and stress manifest themselves in all of us as disorders of our involuntary nervous system, the system over which we have no control. Rapid breathing, a fast pulse, indigestion and irritable bowel syndrome are all examples of the physical effects of anxiety. According to the philosophy of yoga, breathing is central to all these physical effects so this therapeutic discipline concentrates on correct breathing exercises to bring about physical harmony in the body. Yoga breathing exercises teach practitioners to use all of their lungs, not just the upper third, and to use all of the respiratory muscles involved in expanding the chest. As a result, oxygenation of the blood is improved, the involuntary nervous system is stimulated, the circulation boosted and energy and vitality enhanced. Stretching and meditation are often performed at the same time as the breathing exercises.

Based on ancient yogic beliefs, the aim of the treatment is to increase the flow of vital energy or 'prana' which, just as the Chi of ancient Chinese medicine flows along 'meridians', flows along equivalent energy channels called 'nadis'. Yogic tradition pinpoints seven major points of concentrated energy ('chakras') that can be enhanced through yoga. They are found at the crown of the head, the throat, the solar plexus, the spine, the centre of the forehead (the brow chakra or third eye), the heart and the navel. Each chakra, like the Chinese acupressure points, has positive and negative qualities, and can be deliberately stimulated or sedated in order to alter the balance of activity of the central nervous system.

Is yoga effective?

No therapy could survive 5,000 years unless it were hugely beneficial and, anecdotally, there is no doubt that yoga helps millions of people worldwide. There is also a great deal of scientific evidence that yoga has a valuable place as a form of complementary treatment. A research paper published in 1985 in the *British Medical Journal* showed that the regular practice of yoga by asthmatic patients could reduce the number of attacks they experienced and cut down the dosage of drugs needed to control their symptoms. More recently, a paper in the *Journal of Rheumatology* suggested that patients with arthritis of the hands could derive a significant improvement in manual dexterity after two months, with the additional benefit of experiencing less pain. Other studies have shown yoga to be of benefit to those with back pain and anxiety and other stress-related conditions such as palpitations, high blood pressure and stress. It has even been used to great effect in NHS hospitals and hospices for the terminally ill, and in the home environment for patients with those infamously chronic disorders that orthodox medicine is often so ineffective at treating, such as ME (myalgic encephalomyelitis) and emphysema. Much of the work carried out on the therapeutic effect of yoga has been performed by the Yoga Biomedical Trust whose trained practitioners specifically tailor yoga therapy to their individual patients.

What form might the treatment take?

Although it is theoretically possible to learn yoga postures through reading a book or watching a video, this is far from ideal, and the best way is to join a class and be shown exactly what to do. The postures adopted are very precise and usually performed in a specific sequence with the aim of working all the major muscle groups in a logical order to promote good circulation and achieve full relaxation. These postures, or 'asanas', can be adopted at any age and in any state of health, although postures should never be held if they are uncomfortable, and there should be no strain and no tension or hurry.

Usually between 10 and 20 people turn up for a class, which may last between one and two hours. If new to a class, you should let the teacher know if you have any ailments or disabilities so that exercises can be tailored to your individual needs. For some medical problems, one-to-one sessions may be required. It is best to wear loose-fitting clothes, such as a tracksuit, and most people go barefoot. Exercises are performed on comfortable rubber mats, often provided by the class.

By way of warm up, breathing control will be practised first, followed by some initial exercises to stretch the muscles. Later, up to 20 more specific exercises will be adopted in positions for which you stand, sit, kneel or lie, either on the front or back. Often exercises are complementary, in that they work in opposition to one another, and therefore exercise every possible muscle and its antagonist in the body. By way of example, the stomach muscles are antagonistic to the back muscles, the biceps to the triceps, the hamstring to the quadriceps, and so on. Some asanas are purely stretching exercises, for example to extend the spine, and others work on the internal organs in much the same way as acupuncture stimulates the pressure points. Postural exercises are practised in conjunction with correct breathing and relaxation, and most sessions end with deep relaxation exercises and a period of reflection and meditation.

Regular practitioners make yoga part of their everyday activity and use it as a preventative form of therapy, but even new recruits can sometimes benefit from their very first session. After it, many find their general movement lighter and more easy, and the quality of their sleep deeper and more restful.

What problems are helped by yoga?

Yoga can be highly beneficial in treating both physical and psychological disorders. It increases suppleness and muscle tone, so it is of enormous benefit in treating back pain, and many people who have been failed by more orthodox therapies have become disciples of yoga for life as a result of their positive experiences with its practice. Patients with respiratory ailments, such as asthma, hay fever, bronchitis, colds, coughs and sinusitis, and asthma in particular, seem to benefit from its use. Digestive complaints such as irritable bowel syndrome, ulcers and heartburn also respond well. Yoga is therapeutic in all kinds of disability, too, as it is far too easy for muscles to become even weaker when inactivity and disuse affects them. Yoga can teach disabled people to become more aware of their musculo-skeletal system, and mobility can be improved by the regular practice of yoga. The Yoga For Health Foundation is particularly enthusiastic about using this form of complementary therapy in patients with chronic neurological conditions such as multiple sclerosis, muscular dystrophy and other neuro-muscular diseases which are at great risk of being neglected by other medical therapists. For the general population, common ailments which respond well to yoga include anxiety, tension and depression, and all those stress-related conditions such as high blood pressure, indigestion, insomnia, palpitations, poor concentration, lack of confidence and tremor.

Is it safe?

Yoga is essentially safe for people of any age and in any state of health. However, the form the therapy takes should be tailored to people's individual needs, because although exercises can be found to suit everyone, more vigorous types (such as 'ashtanga') which might be appropriate for the young and healthy, might not be for the elderly or osteo-arthritic. In order to achieve mental clarity and inner peace, there must be no strain and no apprehension, and although yoga should never be unchallenging, it should nevertheless put no undue strain on whoever uses it.

How can I find a yoga class?

Most people who enjoy yoga go to classes run by the local community, or to private health centres and sports clubs. Some companies have even set up lunch-time yoga sessions to keep their staff happy and to help employees overcome stress, muscle tension and back problems. Teachers should be members of the British Wheel of Yoga or the Iyengar Yoga Institute. For those people with specific medical disorders, such as chronic and severe backache or asthma, one-to-one sessions can be obtained through contacting the specifically trained therapists of the Yoga Biomedical Trust. They are happy to teach individuals, and they also run classes for small groups of like-minded people.

How much will it cost?

For a lucky few, it is possible to obtain yoga therapy on the NHS following referral by your GP if the local Family Health Services Association has made this possible. Generally, however, sessions are privately funded, costing up to £30 an hour for treatment on a one-to-one basis, or about £10 for a class lasting an hour and a half. Cheaper sessions might be found in larger local authority-run classes, for which just a few pounds may be all that is asked.

The sceptic's view

The hardened sceptic with entrenched views would doubt that

yoga achieves very much at all. There is no evidence that it reduces the incidence of serious diseases like cancer, multiple sclerosis or rheumatoid arthritis, though the sceptic might be prepared to admit it helps some people to breathe properly and can do no harm, but that is about as much as he would concede. To the sceptic, yoga might appear to be nothing more than a fashionable and fanciful time-wasting exercise.

The therapist's view

'It is very rewarding to introduce people to yoga because even after one or two sessions they can begin to experience some of the benefits. Often back pain is eased and stiff joints begin to loosen up. As students begin to be more in touch with their bodies, there is an increase of self-confidence. As they learn relaxation to find some inner stillness, a sense of well-being and a freedom from anxiety is often experienced.

'I like to think that yoga can help to restore people to their natural state of health and happiness.'

Judith Hayes

The patient's view

'I joined a yoga class as middle age approached and I could no longer ignore painful joints and a recurring back problem. Both these complaints ruled out more strenuous forms of exercise. Now after nearly three years, I feel physically so much better; practising yoga gives me an overall sense of well-being, my joints are no longer painful and the back is not a problem.

'I like the calm, non-competitive way in which the postures and exercises are performed. The yoga breathing and relaxation help me to cope with stressful situations and keep the blood pressure in check.'

Margaret O'Malley

Useful Addresses

General

British Complementary Medicine Association
9 Soar Lane
Leicester LE3 5DE
Tel: 0116 242 5406

British Register of Complementary Practitioners
PO Box 194
London SE16 1QZ
Tel: 0171 237 5165

Council for Complementary and Alternative Medicine
Park House
206–208 Latimer Road
London W10 6RE
Tel: 0181 968 3862

The Hale Clinic
7 Park Crescent
London W1N 3HE
Tel: 0171 631 0156

Institute for Complementary Medicines
(operating the British Register of Complementary Practitioners)
PO Box 194
London SE16 1QZ
Tel: 0171 237 5165

The Research Council for Complementary Medicine
60 Great Ormond Street
London WClN 3JF
Tel: 0171 833 8897

Governing and Advisory Bodies

Acupuncture

British Acupuncture Council
Park House
206–208 Latimer Road
LondonW10 6RE
Tel: 0181 964 0222

British Medical Acupuncture Society
Newton House
Newton Lane
Lower Whitley
Warrington
Cheshire WA4 4JA
Tel: 01925 730727

Alexander Technique

Society of Teachers of the Alexander Technique
20 London House
266 Fulham Road
London SW10 9EL
Tel: 0171 351 0828

Aromatherapy

Aromatherapy Organizations Council
3 Latymer Close
Braybrooke
Market Harborough
Leicester LE16 8LN
Tel: 01858 434242

Art Psychotherapy

Association of Drama Therapists
4 Funnydale Villas
Durlston Road
Swanage
Dorset BN19 2HY

British Association of Art Therapists
11a Richmond Road
Brighton
Sussex BN2 3RL

British Society for Music Therapy
25 Rosslyn Avenue
East Barnet EN4 8DH

Autogenic Training

British Association for Autogenic Training and Therapy (BAFATT)
Heath Cottage
Pitch Hill
Ewhurst
Surrey GU6 7NP
Send a s.a.e. for information

Ayurvedic Medicine

Ayurvedic Medical Association UK
17 Bromham Mill
Gilford Park
Milton Keynes MK14 5KP
Tel: 01908 617089

Bach Flower Remedies

The Edward Bach Centre
Mount Vernon
Sotwell
Wallingford
Oxon OX10 0OZ
Tel: 01491 834678

Chinese Herbal Medicine

Register of Chinese Herbal Medicine
PO Box 400
Wembley
Middlesex HA9 9NE
Tel: 0181 904 1347

Chiropractic

British Association for Applied Chiropractic
The Old Post Office
Cherry Street
Stratton Audley
Bicester OX6 9BA

British Chiropractic Association
Equity House
29 Whitley Street
Reading RG1 1QB
Tel: 0118 950 5950

The McTimoney Chiropractic Association
21 High Street
Eynsham
Oxon OX8 1HE
Send a s.a.e. and £1. 50 for a register of practitioners

Scottish Chiropractic Association
30 Roseburn Place
Edinburgh EH12 5NX
Tel: 0131 346 7500

Colonic Hydrotherapy

Colonic International Association
16 Englands Lane
London NW3 4TG
Tel: 0171 483 1593

Colour Therapy

International Association for Colour Therapy
PO Box 3688
London SW13 ONX
Tel: 0181 878 5276

Crystal Therapy

Affiliation of Crystal Healing Organizations
46 Lower Green Road
Esher
Surrey KT10 8HD
Tel: 0181 398 7252

Herbal Medicine

National Institute of Medical Herbalists
56 Longbrook Street
Exeter EX4 6AH
Tel: 01392 426022

Homeopathy

Society of Homeopaths
2 Artizan Road
Northampton NNl 4HU
Tel: 01604 621400

Hypnotherapy

British Society of Experimental and Clinical Hypnosis
c/o Dept. of Psychology
Grimsby General Hospital
Scartle Road
Grimsby DN33 2BA
Tel: 01472 879238

British Society of Medical and Dental Hypnosis
17 Keppel View Road
Kimberworth
Rotherham S61 2AR
Tel: 01709 554558

Iridology

Guild of Naturopathic Iridologists
94 Grosvenor Road
London SW1V 3LF
Tel: 0171 834 3579

International Association of Clinical Iridologists
853 Finchley Road
London NW11 8LX

Macrobiotics

The Kushi Institute
PO Box 7
Becket
MA 01233
USA
Tel: 413 623 5741

Massage Therapy

British Massage Therapy Council
Greenbank House
65a Adelphi Street
Preston PR1 7BH
Tel: 01772 881063

Massage Therapy Institure of Great Britain
PO Box 27/26
London NW2 4NR
Tel: 0181 208 1607

Meditation

Friends of the Western Buddhist Order
London Buddhist Centre
51 Roman Road
London E2 0HU
Tel: 0181 981 1225

School of Meditation
158 Holland Park Avenue
London W11 4UH
Tel: 0171 603 6116

Transcendental Meditation
Freepost
London SW1P 4YY
Tel: 0990 143733

Naturopathy

The General Council and Register of Naturopaths
6 Netherhall Gardens
London NW3 5RR
Tel: 0171 435 8728

Nutritional Therapy

Society for the Promotion of Nutritional Therapy
PO Box 47
Heathfield
East Sussex TN21 8ZX
Tel: O1435 867007

Women's Nutritional Advisory Service
PO Box 268
Lewes
East Sussex BN7 2QN
Tel: 01273 487366

Osteopathy

Osteopathic Information Service
PO Box 2074
Reading
Berkshire RG1 4YR
Tel: 01491 875255

Radionics

The Confederation of Radionic and Radiothesic Organizations
c/o The Maperton Trust
Wincanton
Somerset BA9 8EH
Tel: 01963 36251

The Radionic Association
Baerlein House
Goose Green
Deddington
Banbury
Oxon OX15 0SZ

Reflexology

Association of Reflexologists
Flat 6
Sillwood Mansions
Sillwood Place
Brighton BNl 2LH
Tel: 01273 771061

British Reflexology Association
Monks Orchard
Whitbourne
Worcester WR6 5RB
Tel: 01886 821207

Shiatsu

The Shiatsu Society of Great Britain
5 Foxcote
Wokingham
Berkshire RGl1 3PG
Tel: 01189 730836

Spiritual Healing

The National Federation of Spiritual Healers
Old Manor Farm Studio
Church Street
Sunbury-on-Thames
Middlesex TW16 6RG
Tel: 0891 616080

T'ai Chi

T'ai Chi Union for Great Britain
102 Felsham Road
London SW15 1DQ
Tel: 0171 352 7716

Yoga

British Wheel of Yoga
1 Hamilton Place
Boston Road
Sleaford
Lincolnshire NG34 7ES
Tel: 01529 306851

The Iyengar Yoga Institute
233a Randolf Avenue
London W9 1NL
Tel: 0171 624 3080

Index

Figures in italics refer to tables; those in bold refer to main references to complementary therapies.